COMPLETE SKIN AND HAIR CARE PROGRAM FOR THE ACTIVE MAN

By

M.J. Saffon

with

Charles Francisco

New Century Publishers, Inc.

Library of Congress Cataloging-in-Publication Data

Saffon, M.J.
  Complete skin and hair care program for the active man.

  1. Skin — Care and hygiene.   2. Hair — Care and hygiene. 3. Grooming for men.   I. Francisco, Charles.   II. Title.
RL87.S24   1986   646.7′26   86-8517
ISBN 0-8329-0420-1

Table of Contents

Introduction

At Last! A No-Frills Skin Care Program for the Active Man

During more than twenty-five years of helping the rich and famous—both men and women—improve the health and attractiveness of their skin and hair, I have been deeply disturbed by the self-destructive attitude of most men. They have demonstrated a paranoid reluctance to admit that they care about their appearance. They have been willing to keep themselves neatly groomed, spend money on good tailoring, and so on, but anything more than that— forget it!

This book is proof of my faith that such backward thinking has changed for the better. Wives have told me they have caught their husbands peeking into my best-sellers for women, hoping to find something useful for their own problems. Unfortunately, that doesn't work. There may be minor differences in the physiological composition of male and female skin, but there are monumental differences in how men and women view such a private subject.

1

Androgyny Is Dead—*Vive la Difference*

The program of skin and hair care outlined in this book was created specifically for *men*. The last thing I wanted to do was write a woman's book with a man's title! Something all of us want—in our love lives, on the athletic field, or at work—is a feeling of *control*. With the social upheavals of recent years, gaining control of our destinies is a worthwhile ambition which is becoming more and more elusive.

You Can Control the Way You Look

An active man finally has a real choice about maintaining his youthful good looks. It's a choice he can live with because it demonstrates his common sense rather than a fanciful male ego. Millions of us have learned to care for our bodies for cosmetic as well as health reasons. We now have the same option when it comes to our faces—and it's about time! Look at it this way—you may respect the elderly jogger who has the stamina and muscle tone of a younger man, but if his hair is scraggly and his face has the nooks and crannies of an English muffin, he's still an old man to you, to the woman in his life, and to his employer.

This book deals exclusively with men's problems. It reveals sound methods, most of which you can use in the privacy of your own home, to correct embarrassing problems that have plagued men for centuries. It also analyzes, in a no-nonsense manner, the latest developments in scientific research that have been successful in remedying inherited skin and hair problems that were once thought to be incurable. For the first time, you will know the truth about:

- Male pattern baldness
- Acne, acne scarring
- Five o'clock shadow
- Dandruff
- Ingrown hairs
- Age spots

- Minoxidil, other hair restorers
- Eye bags
- Turkey neck
- Shaving rash
- Broken capillaries
- Sportsman's face
- Dehydration
- Oily skin and hair

These and scores of other skin and hair topics—for men only—are thoroughly examined. The approach is light-hearted, but the aim is totally serious. In short, this book offers a genuine program rather than a series of idle promises.

Your Face Is Your Calling Card

Looking as good as you possibly can—for business and personal reasons—is too important to be taken lightly. We all have to face the reality that every part of the body is going to endure some degree of deterioration with the passage of time. Women fight the encroachment of age by taking special care of their skin and disguising their shortcomings with makeup. Women have politely tried to keep our spirits up but have only succeeded in encouraging the deterioration with their insistence that "some men look more distinguished with a few character lines in their faces."

We have to ignore that flattery. Let's save the "distinguished look" for our seventies. Proper care can't begin too early. The reality is that skin care has nothing to do with gender. Biologically, an All-Pro linebacker comes equipped with skin that is just about as delicate as that of his wife. The primary difference lies in the fact that men have more active hair follicles which enable us to grow beards. Environmental factors—outdoor sports, the workplace—give most of us skin that is a bit thicker than a woman's. Otherwise, your skin and that of your best girl are biologically identical. Let's close this gender gap on a *man's* terms. This book—written by a man for a man—will let you do exactly that.

1

Your Skin:
An Owner's Manual

When I was a little kid, I was crazy about an old song that said, "It ain't no sin to take off your skin and dance around in your bones." Those of us free of serious problems in adolescence were content to think of skin in that offhand manner. It was little more than the outer wrapping that kept all our internal parts from tumbling onto the deck. Not even the most perfect specimen among us can afford to retain that carefree attitude once he reaches his twenties.

In today's super-competitive society, the appearance of the skin on a man's face and the hair on his head takes on increasing importance with each passing year.

Every man starts worrying about the foliage atop his head from the first moment he runs a comb through it and finds that too much of it has left his scalp and taken up residence in the teeth of that comb. We don't give our faces equal time. Traditionally, most of us have been too busy and too "macho." We make the serious error of saying, like Scarlett O'Hara, "I'll worry about that tomorrow." The vital decision to begin an effective skin care program should be approached with the intensity of a baseball player starting the seventh game of a World Series: there is no tomorrow!

Skin: What It Is and How It Works

The skin is the largest organ in your body and also one of the most complex. It is extremely vulnerable to serious damage brought on by neglect and inadequate protection against all manner of environmental pollutants. The skin of your face and neck is the most visible and gets the most abuse, but there's approximately twenty-one square feet of skin covering your entire body. Let's examine skin in general terms to appreciate its nature, its needs, and its complexity.

One square inch of skin contains:

- 19,500,000 cells
- 95–100 oil glands
- 650 sweat glands
- 78 nerves
- 1,300 nerve endings to record pain
- 19,500 sensory cells at ends of nerve fibers
- 78 sensory elements for heat
- 13 sensory elements for cold
- 160–165 pressure elements for touch sense
- 19–20 blood vessels
- 65 hairs and muscles

I've bored you with all of these technical details to impress you with the fact that we're going to be discussing an extremely complex organism. Your face certainly deserves more than a daily scrubbing and shaving. In addition to creating an instant impression on those who view you—too zitty, too oily, too wrinkled, too old —the skin serves a number of all-important functions that affect your entire body. The skin is a breathing organ that helps regulate the body's temperature, acts as a shield to protect the chemical composition of the blood from harmful alkalies and gases, and aids in the elimination of wastes through perspiration. And the nerve endings of the skin are the very first contact points on the complex communication system to the brain. Any sound program to benefit your individual skin must be preceded by a general working knowledge of the male skin.

1. Epidermis
2. Dermis
3. Hypodermis

These labels identify the three primary layers of every man's skin. Everything you do, or don't do, to these layers is going to affect your appearance. Obviously, it's important that you understand their functions. Consider this section your owner's manual, an informal guide to what skin is and how it works.

The Epidermis

The epidermis is the only part of the skin we see. This is the outermost layer which was designed to take a constant daily battering from the elements. However, it is not indestructible. Because it shows, it has been the only part of the skin that most of us have given even elementary care. We washed it, we shaved it, and that was it. Fortunately, in the big picture, the epidermis may be the least important skin component despite its high visibility. It endures the most punishment and has been designed to be an entirely temporary covering. The epidermis is composed of many fine layers of skin cells that nature automatically replaces about every four weeks.

> *Question*: If this is the case, why bother with it?
> *Answer*:   We ain't peeling an orange here, brother!

That frivolous answer was meant to demonstrate that, in this regard, old Adam and Eve were not as lucky as the serpent. Human skin does not come off in a nice even layer like the skin of a snake. The keratinized—or dead—cells are shed in a helter-skelter manner that can wreak real havoc on the skin of your face. The dead cells don't fall away beautifully like a snowstorm. Their exit can be more closely compared to a mudslide. Making certain that the mudslide is cleared away is one of our first duties. Washing your face in the usual manner won't do it! Men have been kept in the dark about this matter for much too long. It's time to take control. The only way we can keep the facial layer of epidermis from looking dead and scaly is by exercising direct, knowledgeable control over its maintenance.

If you have ever taken a really close-up look at your face in a magnified shaving mirror, you have probably noticed the pores in your skin. The sizes of these pores differ in people, depending on the individual skin types we'll discuss later, but all pores become temporarily larger when exposed to heat. It's a common mistake to regard pores as sweat glands when they are actually sebaceous glands, or oil ducts, which help to keep the epidermis lubricated. The amount of oil produced by these glands has a tremendous bearing on the health and appearance of your face.

Keeping this facial lubricant at a proper level and learning to clear away dead skin cells can erase clogged pores and a host of problems. These sebaceous glands produce the oil that is part of something called the natural moisturizing factor. It is this NMF that gives us the unwrinkled, pliable skin of our youth. Age begins to rob us of some of these natural benefits, even before we reach twenty-five. We will learn how to overcome this potential loss in the uncomplicated but invaluable steps that I will outline later in this book.

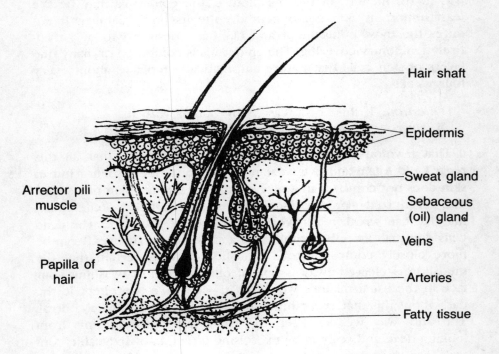

Skin

The Dermis

You can't see it, but the layer of skin called the dermis is more important than the epidermis in the long-term appearance of your face. Most of the elements contained in a square inch of skin, which I listed earlier, reside in the dermis. The dermis is more protected than the epidermis because it acts as its support system. The appearance of the outer skin of your face will ultimately be determined by the condition of your dermis, because that is its primary source of nourishment. Conversely, improper care of your epidermis is going to foul up the health of your dermis and what lies under it.

Collagen is a word you have probably heard, usually as an ingredient in the more expensive skin care products for women. Actually, the dermis of both men and women is composed primarily of collagen. Collagen is a fibrous protein surrounding the blood capillaries that supply the skin with oxygen, the lymph vessels, the nerves and nerve endings, and the hair follicles. The dermis is also the seat of the oil and sweat glands that keep the skin supple and rid it of wastes.

It is the fibrous collagen of the dermis that gives our facial skin its elasticity. Keeping the collagen healthy is an important task because nearly all permanent damage to the facial skin results from the effects of neglect, abuse, and age on the dermis. Age will always collect its toll, but we can slow down its effect through proper care.

Even more discouraging to those past forty is the sad fact that damage to the dermis cannot be corrected. However, the sooner you abandon damaging practices, the more likely you are to be able to maintain a healthy and youthful appearance. Normal aging and the ultraviolet rays of the sun are the collagen's greatest enemies. We can fight these enemies by combining a minimum of time with a maximum of what our grandfathers called old-fashioned horse sense.

The Hypodermis

Beneath the dermis is the final major component of the skin, called the hypodermis. The hypodermis is a layer of fatty connective tissue that literally acts as a cushion for the dermis. Because it is the deepest skin layer, there is little we can do on the surface to protect it. However, all is not lost. I will give you a program of exercise that will definitely help the situation. A proper diet can also forestall the loss of the fatty tissue—the substance that gives the face its natural contours—and bring an altered appearance in the September of our years.

Wrap Up

If you've followed me closely to this point, you can relax with the knowledge that I've been about as dryly scientific as I intend to get. What I have laid out in these opening pages are a few specifics about the actual physiological composition of the skin. I simply wanted to bring home the point that this outer covering of ours is a far more fragile substance than we have been taught to think it is.

The fragility I'm talking about has nothing whatever to do with masculinity or femininity. It has everything to do with the face that was issued to you. You can't trade it in for a newer model. It's the only one you're ever going to have, unless you're prepared for extensive plastic surgery. Keeping it in good shape can be a rewarding experience.

> *Rule*: Like a *grand vin* that accompanies a sumptuous
> *entree*, your face should receive the attention it
> deserves.

Although they're made of the same stuff, no two skins are identical. With your help, I can give you excellent advice for your individual skin care program without the necessity of seeing you in person. Together, through the pages of this book, we'll work out a program individually tailored to your face, your schedule, and your lifestyle. We'll take it one step—or chapter—at a time.

2

Discovering Your
Skin Type

Question: If, as you say, the skin of men and women is
almost identical, what is this business about
skin types?

As I mentioned in the first chapter, all skin is composed of the same
basic elements. However, these elements do not perform in the
same manner for all people, male or female. Age, heredity, and a
number of other factors come into play to give the lie to the
glorious words of the Preamble to the U.S. Constitution insofar as
the skin and hair are concerned. In that regard, all men are not
created entirely equal. For the purpose of clarification, skin specialists have categorized the general skin types.

By using the words *extra* or *super*, it's possible to come up with
a long list of perfectly legitimate skin types. I feel such hyperbole
only adds to the confusion. Our only goal in this book is to help
you find ways to effect changes in your skin, if that is desirable.
Identifying your present type and its problems is the first serious
step you will take toward making your own skin healthy and hand-
some. To add further confusion to this situation, what most doctors
call normal skin is so rare it's almost nonexistent, particularly in
men over the age of twenty-five. My goal is to give you the infor-

mation that will help you to make your own skin "normal," despite present problems and chronological age. Here's the categorization that most dermatologists use:

1. Normal
2. Oily
3. Dry
4. Dehydrated/aging
5. Combination

You can certainly identify your skin, to one degree or another, under one of these general headings. Each of these skin types has particular problems that must be approached in specific ways. Understanding each skin type, even those that don't match yours at the moment, will make it easier for you to recognize and correct flaws in your own situation.

Normal Skin

This rarest blessing belongs to those who have voted in perhaps just two presidential elections. So-called normal skin is exactly what all of us want to have because all the pumps are working to perfection. In other words, if you have normal skin, it is both healthy and balanced, with the oil glands supplying just enough sebum to keep your epidermis well lubricated without clogging the pores.

Face it—you have a state-of-the-art covering. Your pores are of uniform size and barely visible, and the skin is receiving an ample supply of blood and other nutrients from the dermis. Because all of the components are functioning to perfection, the man with normal skin has far less reason to anticipate immediate problems with blemishes and wrinkles. If all this luxury describes the skin of your face, take a deep breath and count yourself among the blessed. But do not relax!

Those who have normal skin simply cannot afford to take it for granted. Without proper care, the best skin will fade. The steady passage of time—not to mention exposing the face to the elements—is going to cause the anointed eventually to join the rest of us. Those lucky enough to have been born with normal skin have been given a head start, but no one gets a lifetime guarantee. Only proper maintenance will keep any skin healthy and youthful.

Oily Skin

This is the skin problem that plagues so many during puberty. Some of us outgrow it in our early twenties, many don't. With this skin type, the oil glands produce an overabundance of sebum, the colorless and odorless substance that keeps the skin moisturized. At first glance that would seem to be a decided plus, but problems arise because the epidermis insists on its process of continued renewal.

A disadvantage for men with oily skin is that the pores are enlarged and uneven. When the dead cells of the epidermis detach themselves, the surplus oil often causes them to stick to the skin's surface, clogging the pores. This, in turn, produces blackheads and other unpleasant eruptions.

Obviously, the need here is to rid the skin's surface of excess oil in order to keep the pores from clogging and to keep the epidermis in a well-balanced state. Getting rid of excess oil would seem to be a rather easy task for anyone who has ever mopped a greasy kitchen floor. However, *well-balanced* is the key word here. This is not a simple matter of washing the face repeatedly with a strong detergent or using drying agents. That can do as much harm as good in the long run.

There are decided disadvantages in having oily skin, but the story is certainly not all bad. If you have naturally oily skin, the time will come when you'll be luckier than others, once you get the problem under control. Your hard-working sebaceous glands are keeping your face naturally well lubricated, and that means your skin will be far less likely to develop wrinkles. If you make a serious effort to practice my complete skin care program—to the point where you get those runaway oil ducts under control—you'll be far less likely to show signs of aging. Before long, you'll be able to flash a sympathetic smile at the uninformed man who entered his productive years with so-called normal skin.

Dry Skin

Reverse the above situation and you have dry skin. Men with dry skin have oil glands that fail to produce enough sebum to keep the skin properly lubricated. Like Arab shieks, our job is to get those wells pumping. A bad case of dry skin presents us with a whole new set of problems.

Dry skin lacks lubrication and will become flaky. It will have very small pores, and it will also be inclined to develop wrinkles much more quickly. Men with severely dried skin are leaving themselves open to increasing problems, including dehydration.

On the other hand, a man with dry skin will be less inclined to suffer from blackheads and other skin eruptions. However, he should be especially careful of sunburn and windburn, and he will find that his face becomes easily irritated. The really good news is that dry skin can be brought back to normal with informed care.

Dehydrated/Aging Skin

Although *dry* and *dehydrated* are relatively synonymous words, there are distinct differences in the skin types. Dry skin suffers from a lack of oil, while dehydrated skin endures the exact problem the name implies: it lacks water. Every skin, even if oily, is susceptible to dehydration from time to time. For that matter, the natural aging process causes the skin to dehydrate a bit more with each passing year unless steps are taken to avoid it. That's why we have lumped dehydrated and aging skin together.

The insidious danger lies in the fact that many men have an almost constant case of dehydrated skin without even being aware of the problem. Anything that tends to dehydrate the body—too much booze, crash diets, hormonal imbalance, glandular problems, and too much time in the sun and wind—can cause the face to look much older than the date on your birth certificate would indicate.

The skin of your face, if you have a problem with dehydration, will feel bone dry. It will have a pronounced lack of elasticity, and you will begin to develop a spate of thin lines in the area around the eyes and on the cheeks. The cowboy who "rides the desert wastes" may sell a lot of cigarettes, but the gullies and ravines on his kisser are a telltale mark that he is suffering from dehydrated skin. The decision to have these so-called character lines is strictly yours to make.

Combination Skin

Like they say, you can't take Mother Nature for granted. If you've been thinking while reading this material that parts of your face are oily while others are dry, you have combination skin. Believe me, that isn't what people mean when they talk about having it all. It might be comforting to know that you are not alone.

According to scientific research, nearly 80 percent of all men tested have combination skin. From that point of view, what we call combination skin would seem to be more deserving of the title "normal." However, the lack of normalcy comes because various areas of your face are receiving nourishment in unequal proportions. If you have this problem, it means your facial skin is very badly unbalanced.

In most instances, a man with combination skin will find that he has an excessively oily area that runs across the forehead and down the nose and chin. At the same time, the skin around his eyes, on his cheeks, and on his neck will be unusually dry. This combination of problems means that each area must be cared for separately, but the program I have planned for you will enable you to do this in a very few minutes each day. The results will make the bit of extra effort very worthwhile.

Your Own Skin Type

You now have a working knowledge of the skin. It's time to begin work on your individual program of skin care and maintenance. You can discover your personal skin type on your own without a visit to a skin specialist. Do go if you have some uncommon skin problem. If not, whatever your age or ethnic background, you will recognize your place in one of the skin type groupings we have covered.

The first tool you're going to need is a mirror. We've been taught since birth that prolonged staring into a mirror smacks of vanity, if not narcissism, but we've got to know where we're at before we can move on to a better place. If you don't have a magnified shaving mirror, the few bucks necessary to buy one should be considered a good investment.

Okay, ignore the face and concentrate solely on every area of epidermis that covers it. Look for the signs that indicate the variety of skin types we have mentioned. As a reminder, here's a list of those types and the things that might be noticeable.

Type Casting—Quick Menu

1. *Normal skin*: Barely visible pores, no blackheads or other zits, no heavy lines or wrinkles.
2. *Oily skin*: Large visible pores, excess sheen, rough texture, possible blackheads and blemishes.
3. *Dry skin*: Almost invisible pores, many fine wrinkles, little sheen, possible flakiness.
4. *Dehydrated/aging skin*: No discernible pores, dull color, parchmentlike appearance, dry to the touch.
5. *Combination skin*: Oily sheen on forehead, nose, and chin; dryness and possible wrinkling around eyes and on cheeks and neck.

If you think it's necessary, keep this list near so you can check it against all the signs you read on your own face. Again, I want you to examine your skin as closely as possible. Between close observation in a mirror and your sense of touch, you should be able to get a pretty fair idea of your personal skin type. If you're still confused, stand by.

There's another simple way to pinpoint your skin type, at home in the privacy of your own bathroom. If you have given your face a thorough cleaning before going to sleep, you can conduct this test when you get up in the morning. Otherwise, it's best to do this when you have a bit of free time to spend at home after properly washing your face. The reason for this is that it will take quite a few minutes for your skin to regain its normal acid mantle after a good cleansing.

Making certain your face is really clean is important because we're going to be checking for the presence of sebum and natural moisture rather than a mixture of sweat and grime. We'll talk about the specific types of cleaning agents you should use for your individual skin and the reasons for doing so later. For now, just use the mildest soap available. Your wife or girlfriend will probably have a special soap that she uses on her face—yet another indication that women have been way ahead of us in skin care know-how. Latch on to her soap, or, if she refuses to share it, take some of your own shave cream (unmentholated) and use it as a soap. Wash your face carefully, making certain that you rinse it very thoroughly to remove all traces of the cleanser from the surface of your face. Now you can gather some materials and relax while you wait for your skin to reform its natural acid mantle.

Your tools for this research will be pieces of paper. What we want is paper that will be thin and porous enough to pick up the natural moisture of your skin. Onionskin typing paper, cigarette paper, or even thin brown wrapping paper will do the job. While you're waiting for the skin's natural mantle to return, cut the paper you have selected into strips, an inch or so wide by two to three inches long. Carry on with your normal morning routine for a half-hour or so, and you'll be ready to begin the test, with your skin now back in its usual state. Take one of your pieces of paper and attempt to stick it to the center of your forehead. If you have oily or combination skin and the paper isn't too thick and heavy, it will probably stick. If it doesn't stay there, gently wipe the center of your forehead with it. Now examine the paper to see if it shows an oily spot.

Repeat this process with new strips of paper on each side of the forehead, on the nose, and on the chin. What we're doing, of course, is testing your T zone. The paper will only stick on skin that is excessively oily, but most skin types should show an oil spot after the paper has been rubbed on these usually oily areas. If you get no oily spot at all after testing this T zone, your skin is unusually dry and possibly dehydrated. Check each strip of paper again after a few minutes to make certain that it has not been temporarily stained by perspiration.

Our next move is to test the areas of the face that are normally less oily in all skin types. Again, using new strips of paper, follow the same procedure on the inner and outermost parts of the cheek,

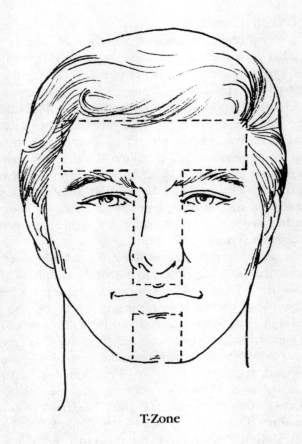

T-Zone

the outer portions of the chin, the jaw line, and the neck. Even if you have oily skin, it's unlikely the paper will stick to any of these areas, so rub each strip gently in an attempt to get an oil stain. The spots should be noticeably lighter because the sebaceous glands do not produce as much sebum in these areas. Here s another quick checklist to help you find your personal skin type using this method.

Paper Proof

1. *Normal skin*: Light paper may stick temporarily to middle of forehead, nose, and center of chin. Oil spots will be subtly present.

2. *Oily skin*: Paper will stick to T zone and inner cheek areas, and the oil spot will be readily apparent, turning paper almost transparent.

3. *Dry/dehydrated skin*: Light paper may not stick anywhere. Oily spot almost nonexistent except on nose.

4. *Combination skin*: Paper may well stick on areas of the T zone, but will show only light oil spot when applied elsewhere.

This procedure seems pretty silly in its simplicity, but you are not required to walk around for hours with pieces of paper stuck to your mug. The paper test can be completed in privacy and takes only a few minutes. It is a completely painless and inexpensive endeavor that has withstood the test of time. More importantly, between the paper test and your own visual and tactile examination, you should now know your individual skin type.

Solving the pH Mystery

Question: I keep seeing ads, especially on TV, talking about something called *pH* and how important it is to the stuff women use on their faces and hair. If there's no big difference between the skin of men and women, how come they need this pH stuff and we don't?

Answer: You do! Advertising about the pH factor is directed primarily at women because they have always been more receptive to information on how to care for their skin and hair.

General information on the pH factor is important to you at this point in my program because it will have a direct bearing on everything you will be doing to return or keep your skin and hair in top-notch condition. The term *pH* is a chemical abbreviation for *potential of hydrogen*, or the balance of hydrogen ions in a substance. In other words, the pH scale will tell us the degree of alkalinity and acidity in a product. Attaining the proper balance between acidity and alkalinity for your personal skin and hair is as important to you as it is to a woman.

The complete skin and hair care regimen outlined in this book makes it unnecessary for you to worry about all the ins and outs of the pH factor. However knowing the basics of the pH factor will be a help when you return from a hard day at the job and discover that you're out of soap, shampoo, after shave, or some other vital product. A quick trip to the corner store to grab just anything off the shelf can lead to a setback in the good effort you've already given to your skin and hair care program. Eventually, whatever you put on your face is going to have some effect on the acid mantle of your skin. That acid mantle is your first and last line of defense.

The pH scale runs from 1 to 14. Water registers at pH 7. That makes water completely neutral in the matter of alkalinity and acidity. Numbers higher than pH 7 indicate a higher degree of alkalinity. Bleach ranges between 12 and 14. Numbers below 7 on the scale tell us that the substance is basically acid. Hydrochloric acid, for example, registers 1 on the pH scale.

Normal, healthy human skin and hair ranges from pH 4.5 to pH 5.5. The preceding sentence is the primary thing you must know about the pH factor, because keeping your skin and hair as biologicaly normal and healthy as possible is the ultimate objective in this program. I know that time is money to you, so I'm not going to waste it by loading you down with a lot of home remedies. You can clean your skin and hair safely and efficiently with commercial products. However, read the labels to make certain you are not purchasing a product that will destroy the natural order of things. Unfortunately, most manufacturers have yet to list specific details about the pH factor on their labels. This shortsightedness is bound to be corrected in the near future as more and more people of both sexes become interested in proper skin care. Look for products that say pH balanced.

I will be giving you the names of specific products that I have tested, appropriate for your skin type, in the next chapter. In general terms, most name-brand soaps and shampoos range from 8 to 9 on the pH scale, placing them well over on the alkaline side of neutral. Since the perfect pH of the skin hovers around 5, this means that many commercial soaps are going to strip away your acid mantle as readily as they remove the dirt and grime from your skin. Unless your occupation or hobby causes your face and hair to get covered in some impossible-to-remove matter, there simply is no reason to use a cleaner that could end up doing as much harm as good. We have to resist the lures of advertising, break our old habits, and use skin and hair products that are appropriate for each of us as individuals. Cleaners that are too alkaline or too acid can cause harm to your outer covering, much as acid rain raises hell with a northern forest.

3

Keep It Clean!

Question: By sheer accident, of course, I have glanced through a few skin care books for women where they were instructed to slap stuff on their faces that seemed more appropriate as part of a fine meal than a cleaning ritual. You're not planning on telling me to do this fruit salad and omelette routine, are you?

Answer: Nope. It takes a man to know that most men aren't going to be that easily led.

If I've made an accurate judgment of your character and lifestyle, you're a busy guy who has neither the time nor the inclination to whip up a batch of home remedies in the kitchen. It is not that I disapprove of such treatments. Some of them can be very effective, especially for a man with extra-sensitive or problem skin. However, if you have some abnormal skin problem, you would be better advised to see a dermatologist rather than relying on this or any other book.

Face Facts

1. Nothing will clean your skin better than a bar of good hard-milled soap.
2. Select a soap that is suitable for your individual skin type.
3. Only those with soap-sensitive or extra-dry skin need to worry about the alkaline pH of soap.
4. The high price of a soap does not necessarily make it better.

Question: You talked earlier about the importance of the pH factor. Aren't you contradicting yourself by telling me to use soap?

Answer: Not at all. We should be aware of the acid mantle of the skin and the necessity of keeping it in good balance. But a good face soap, properly used, will affect the mantle only temporarily, and the resulting cleanliness will allow it to return to normal condition.

Surprisingly, soap has only been around since medieval times. People were just not that concerned with cleanliness in bygone days. Unfortunately, what we know as modern deodorants came along much later. Soap is basically a combination of animal or vegetable fat that has been combined and cooked with a strong alkali. The resultant substance is then cooled and pressed into a bar. We also have modern detergents which serve the same general purpose but are composed of artificial fats or petroleum additives. The advantage of detergents over regular soaps is that they can be less alkaline and less inclined to stick to your skin after washing. The only two drawbacks to soap have to do with its alkaline nature. These minuses are relatively insignificant; they are naturally drying and do clear away bacteria. The thing to remember is not to overdo a good thing.

Although most men are only now beginning to look into the advantages of skin care, the people who manufacture men's grooming products have seen to it that men have an opportunity to buy almost any kind of soap they can imagine. The thing to remember is that high price does not necessarily equate with better performance. It's possible to pay more than eight dollars a bar for a special name-brand soap that has been aimed at the men's market, but there is no scientific evidence that it will actually clean your skin any better or with more gentleness than one of the under-a-buck bars you can pick off the shelf of a supermarket. Most such high-priced soaps claim to have undergone rigorous testing that makes them special, but nearly all soaps, whatever the price, have undergone the same process.

> *Question*: Listen, I love the scent of the after shave, cologne, and other products I use (and so do the women in my life). This company also makes a soap. Anything wrong with using it?
>
> *Answer*: Not a thing, as long as you know the soap is right for your skin.

Fragrance is the very least important thing about the soap you select for regular use. In reality, its only effect will be on your psychological well-being and your wallet. The popular and expensive grooming products for men got that way primarily because of their distinctive scents. If you like a scent, good for you. In the case of soap, you are the only one who will be able to smell it, and only while you are washing. Since, as we've said, all soap is drying when left on the skin, it is all-important that we take pains to thoroughly rinse all of the soapy residue off the skin after washing. If you do an adequate job of rinsing, the fragrance of the soap will be gone. From the dollars-and-cents point of view, why pay more for a scent that you should have completely washed away before leaving the bathroom?

> *Question*: What is the big deal about washing? Isn't that something we all learn by the age of three?
>
> *Answer*: True enough. And if getting the daily dirt off our mugs was the only problem we face, there would be no reason for this section of the book. But that isn't good enough for our purposes.

The simple act of washing the face is the first step in any knowledgeable program of good care and maintenance for the skin. Improper or lackadaisical cleaning rivals natural aging and the sun as powerful enemies of the face.

Why We Wash

1. Our mothers forced us.
2. Polite society demands it.

Okay, so I was only joking. However, the fact remains that we should wash our faces for reasons other than avoiding the reputation as the dirtiest kid on the block. Cleanliness may be next to godliness as the old proverb says, but maintaining our best appearance will also enable us to move closer to some heavenly bodies who are far more earthbound—and earthy. In other words, washing your face in this program will do more than simply rid it of dirt.

What Face Washing Should Do

1. Clean the skin.
2. Exfoliate the skin.
3. Stimulate the skin.
4. Restore the balance.

Remember when we were discussing the epidermis, the outer layer of skin that is the only part we actually see? Well, it's important to recall that the epidermis is continually sloughing off dead cells. These dead cells can cause more harm than everyday dirt because they clog the pores and start all kinds of problems unless they're properly removed. Among skin specialists, the removal of these dead cells is called exfoliation or epiabrasion. This process can be done while you are washing your face. You will be stimulating and moisturizing your facial skin at the same time, and the proper balance of your acid mantle will be restored by the time you're ready to greet your colleagues.

Choosing a Soap

It is important to choose the correct soap for your personal skin type, but you don't have to hire a private eye or a personal researcher to find it. As I indicated earlier, there are soaps available for every skin type in a wide range of prices. Many of these are made specifically for men and can be found only in the better department stores. If you don't mind spending the money, go for it. On the other hand, I have found that there are readily available soaps that cost far less and do the job equally well.

I am an independent practitioner and do not work for any manufacturer, so I avoid recommending specific name-brand products. However, in order to give you an example of the kinds of cleaners I would recommend in an in-person session, I'll bend that rule a little here. In our earlier listing of the skin types, we came up with several to make it easier for you to identify your own. Now we can break that list down even more, skin that is oily and skin that is dry. When it comes to soap, those are the important determinations.

In this case, skin that tends to be dry, dehydrated, or aging are the most susceptible to damage from the wrong kind of soap because that substance itself is naturally drying. As a general rule, for a man with normal, dry, dehydrated, or aging skin, I would suggest that he try using a bar soap such as Dove or Correct. Both of these are good cleaners and are pH balanced to make certain they will not harm your skin. These types of soap will also serve well on combination skin, unless your T zone is positively oozing oil like a leaky crankcase. If you have oily skin, you will have less need to worry about your specific brand of soap. Again, we're talking about the average oily skin that is not plagued by really severe acne or other major problems. Your job is to remove that excess oil and the dead cells that have clung to your face because of it. You have a wider choice of soaps because you want your skin to be dryer. Two examples you might try are Neutrogena or Cuticura.

Shortcuts

1. In a pinch, don't hesitate to use your wife's special soap. It's sure to be gentle.
2. If you spend much time on the road, buy one of those plastic containers and take your personal soap with you.

Question: I'm a guy who perspires a lot, and I worry about body odor. For that reason, I take at least a shower a day and use a strong deodorant soap. Is it okay if I wash my face with the same soap in the shower?

Answer: If you don't mind a face that smells great but looks awful.

Actually. the flippant answer above is meant to be a reminder that common sense should guide all of our actions—in love, business, and personal grooming. Many deodorant soaps contain an ingredient the chemists call triclocarbon which is designed to kill the odor-causing bacteria on the skin. These ingredients can cause rashes and other problems on sensitive skin, and they were never intended to be used on the face. If you prefer to clean your face when you shower, take your face soap into the shower with you. There are even better reasons to make your face washing a separate exercise, as I'll explain shortly.

When to Wash

Another illustration of the fact that washing the face is not the simple chore we may have imagined it to be is that it is possible for some men to do it too often. To be specific, those who have extremely dry or dehydrated skin could do some damage by overdoing the soap-and-water routine, even when using a soap that is right for their skin. This is particularly true for older men whose sebaceous glands have slowed down in their production of natural oil to lubricate the epidermis. Conversely, it is almost impossible for a younger man with very oily skin to overdo the face-washing routine.

Most men should make a habit of washing the face twice each day. Washing twice a day, with the proper soap and technique, can do nothing but help the skin. You will be removing all of the environmental pollution that affects everything and everyone in today's world. By doing so, you will be diminishing the effects of possible damage by these unknown agents. You will also be accomplishing the aims we listed earlier: exfoliating, stimulating, and restoring the normal acid mantle.

Ideally, the best times for cleaning the face would be first thing in the morning and in the late afternoon or early evening. The face suffers the most outside abuse in the daytime, during waking and working hours. In today's hectic society, when a busy professional often doesn't have the luxury of nine-to-five hours, it's nearly impossible to find the time to do a good job of personal grooming as soon as the day's work is completed. For that reason, we'll take the easiest way out: clean up upon rising and before retiring.

The foregoing is intended only as a guideline. If you have a job that requires the kind of physical endeavor that leaves you unfit for polite company, by all means don't wait until bedtime. If you make regular visits to a gym or health club, give your face a workout along with your shower. Men with very oily skin could benefit from a thorough washing whenever they feel the need, especially during the hot months. On the other end of the scale, men with very dry or dehydrated skin must guard against overdoing it, especially during the colder months when everyone's skin becomes dryer.

Water Temperature

There was a time when your mother wouldn't even think of washing your dirty blue jeans without using strong soap and very hot water. That has changed for the better, and, fortunately, so have our ideas about the uses of water on our faces. As I hinted earlier, even the temperature of the air can have a great effect on the condition of the skin. With the improved soaps available today, there is no need to use very hot water to do a good job of cleaning—on clothing or skin. Any athlete knows that heat causes muscles to relax. By the same token, an overuse of heat on the face can induce long-term damage to the facial muscles, causing a gradual breakdown of the dermis and hypodermis. This can lead to sagging facial contours.

Heavy use of very hot water on the skin also causes the pores to open more than necessary, and this robs the skin of its natural moisture. This will have relatively little effect on young men with oily skin, but it will work against the general good of the skin as we grow older. The dermis simply provides less oil and moisture as we age. Men with dry or dehydrated skin and most men past thirty should spend less time in hot showers and tub baths. Settle for cooler water when bathing, and certainly shun very hot water when washing the face.

Rule: Water should be lukewarm for washing the face, regardless of skin type.

Exfoliating

It sounds a bit like clearing a jungle, doesn't it? What it boils down to in common language is simply working a little harder to get the dead skin cells off the face to prevent their clogging the pores. Washing the face with a good soap and rinsing thoroughly will do a big part of the job, but many of us need a little extra effort. There are several commercial products available specifically for epiabrasion or exfoliation. One is a textured polyester sponge, and another is a more expensive item made with natural fibers and called a loofah. Both of these aids can be found in most drug stores.

I have found that two items you probably already have on hand will work just as well for most men. One is the common terry washcloth, and the other is a shaving brush. Exfoliation is simply scrubbing the skin to loosen the dead cells. A washcloth, along with the proper soap, will do a fine job. A word of caution: be sure to use fresh washcloths as often as possible because they can become excellent devices for spreading infection. There is also the possibility that the texture of the washcloth, along with overvigorous rubbing, will prove to be too rough for those with severe acne or sensitive and badly dehydrated skin.

My favorite tool for exfoliating, and the one that should be comfortable for anyone, is the natural-bristle shaving brush. The shaving brush has pretty much gone out of favor with the advent of aerosol foams and the like, and I'll go into great detail about shaving in the next chapter. But I would advise anyone to invest in a good shaving brush that can be used for a variety of purposes. Make certain that you use a brush with natural fibers.

Shaving Brush Exfoliation

1. Rinse the face thoroughly with lukewarm water.
2. Apply generous amount of soap to every portion of the face.
3. Take a clean natural-fiber shaving brush and work soap into a

lather, going over ever inch of the face in small circular motions.

4. Rinse carefully until all traces of soap residue disappear.

You will find that shaving brush exfoliating will be a pleasant and worthwhile endeavor. The natural bristles are tough enough to do a good job of epiabrasion, and yet they should not prove to be an irritant even to the most sensitive skin.

Rinsing

Rule: Rinsing the soap off the skin should be considered as important as applying it.

No matter how rushed you may be, don't settle for a few quick splashes of water on the face after you have finished washing. Remember, soap itself is drying. Take time to wash away every bit of the soap that has been on your skin. Now that you've decided to get into the race, why not go for the gold?

I doubt that you've read anything in this section that you will find particularly earthshaking, but I'm also assuming that you've been around long enough to appreciate the fact that attention to detail gets the job done. This face-cleaning regimen is only your first simple step toward achieving healthier, better-looking skin.

Face Cleaning—Quick Menu

1. Choose a hard-milled bar soap appropriate to your skin type.
2. Do not use deodorant soap on the face.
3. Scented soaps serve no purpose.
4. Make a habit of A.M. and P.M. washings.
5. Use lukewarm water for washing the face.
6. Use generous amounts of the appropriate soap.
7. Exfoliate the skin—scrub—with the soap.
8. A natural-bristle shaving brush is the best tool for exfoliating.
9. Rinse carefully until soap film vanishes.

4

The Do's and Don'ts of Shaving

Returning to the classic men vs. women theme, the primary difference between the skin on your face and that on the face of a women is that yours grows copious amounts of facial hair. This was probably an enormous source of pride for you when the first few scraggly whiskers began to sprout way back when, but the regular shaving routine can become an irritating, tedious chore when you've done it for a few years.

Yet those minutes we spend removing the most burdensome byproduct of our testosterone give us a built-in advantage over women in terms of good skin care. Women using makeup run the risk of putting things on their skin that can do it harm. Men, by removing the omnipresent stubble, have a macho means of simultaneously improving our skins. Unfortunately, most men have always considered shaving a drudgery rather than an opportunity. In this section we'll examine improved methods of shaving that will do more than scratch the surface of enlightened skin care.

Question: I started shaving at the age of fourteen when my chin began to look like the surface of a new tennis ball. After twenty-two years of this

> daily nonsense, do you really think you can
> teach me anything new about shaving?

I'll begin my answer to that question by asking one of my own. Who taught you the technique of shaving in the first place? Chances are, like most of us, you either leaped into adolescent experimentation as early proof of your approaching manhood, or you turned to your father for expert advice. Good old Dad would never give you a bum steer deliberately, but his expertise probably came from his own father years before your birth. Times have changed.

The sad truth of the matter is that almost all men, including barbers, have not kept up with new developments in the art of sensible shaving. No two skins are identical, and shaving should be a highly individual act in the interest of maintaining a smooth, fine-toned face for longer than the duration of the shave. The usual assembly-line scraping we have been conditioned to rely on is not the result of some sinister plot darker than your five o'clock shadow, but rather the fallout of a failure to pass along important new information to the general public. Old habits, especially bad ones, are hard to break. But now that we have supersonic jets, there's little reason to attempt a crossing of the Atlantic in a canoe.

An Old Dad's Tale
(How to Get a Proper Shave)

1. Apply steaming hot water or towels to soften the beard.
2. Cover shaving area liberally with thick foam.
3. Use long, firm strokes, upward for a closer shave.
4. Rinse and cover shaved area with a bracing after-shave lotion.

Contemporary Critique

1. Wrong
2. Wrong
3. Wrong
4. Wrong

We can damage our faces unintentionally in such a routine chore as shaving. Almost all men do shave in a manner similar to that described above. Instead of daily drudgery, I would like you to look at shaving as part of your skin care regimen.

We must refer again to the underlying but all-important skin component called the dermis which we discussed earlier in this book. At the very least, shaving should provide the dermis with the gentle massage it needs to retain the elasticity that enables it to support the thin layers of the epidermis. The materials we use in the process—from blades and lubricants to water and after shave— all have an ability to help or harm the skin of the face. Because we lacked information, most of us have long treated the dermis and the epidermis to a daily boiling, pulling, scraping, and bruising, followed by a sadistic bath in an alcohol-based liquid that further dehydrates the skin and causes it to dispatch urgent messages to the brain that spell out P-A-I-N! Let's pledge to rid ourselves of the stubble in ways that are less agonizing and far more beneficial for the face.

>*Rule*: Always shave in accordance with the special problems and needs of your skin type.

If you happen to be one of the rare young guys blessed with what has been mislabeled normal skin, you could get away with shaving in Old Dad's way—for a time. You have no glaring skin problems, and the outdated shaving method will give you no immediate trouble. However, skin damage is cumulative, and your face will begin reflecting that daily battering as you add a few years.

What's Wrong with Old Dad's Method?

1. Long use of very hot water is harmful to any type of skin. It can cause sebaceous glands in oily skin to work harder and lead to broken blood vessels and further dehydration for those with dry skin.

2. Aerosol foams appear thick and rich, but most of them are mainly water and air bubbles that do little to protect sensitive skin from the pulling and scraping of a razor blade.

3. Firm upward strokes with a blade create all kinds of problems including abrasions, ingrown hairs, and blotchiness.

4. Standard after-shave lotions are primarily alcohol, a powerful drying agent that can bring on skin dehydration, flaking, and early wrinkling.

That brief rundown should help convince you that continued use of the old-fashioned method of shaving will lead to nothing but grief as the years roll by. The minutes you spend in front of your shaving mirror should be a vital part of your determination to keep your skin healthy and youthful. I'll discuss the advantages and disadvantages of the different types of razors later in this chapter. For now, let's assume that you use a regular safety-blade razor. Let us also assume that you have average skin, a combination of dry and oily with no special problems. The following is a daily shaving routine that will keep you looking and feeling much younger than the date on your birth certificate.

Face-Saving Shaving

Step 1. You have already washed and exfoliated the face. Now bathe or shower, using water somewhat warmer than you used on your face.

Step 2. Out of the tub, rinse the face thoroughly again in lukewarm water.

Step 3. Do not dry, but immediately apply a generous amount of a safe shaving cream over the area to be shaved, making certain it is fully protected.

Step 4. Be sure to use a sharp blade and shave in smooth, gentle strokes, following the direction of hair growth. Use long strokes on cheeks and jaw and short strokes near nose and mouth and on the chin. Avoid extra pressure for closeness.

Step 5. Thoroughly rinse the face with lukewarm water after shaving to remove all traces of the shaving cream. Pat face dry with towel.

Step 6. Spray fine water mist on shaved area and cover with invisible men's water-based moisturizer. If scent is desired, use a minute dab of your favorite men's cologne on the neck near each ear.

This is the safest, most comfortable shaving technique for all men, regardless of skin type. Obviously, men with pronounced skin problems should take extra care with the preparations they put on their faces and the type of razors they use. I am not going to claim, as one manufacturer does, that shaving is a "sensuous" experience. It is a chore, but an important one that we can turn to our advantage. Let's put it in perspective.

Bare-Faced Truths

- A dry whisker has the toughness of a copper wire of the same thickness.
- The average beard contains approximately 15,500 hairs.
- Most beards grow about five and a half inches a year, averaging 15/1000 of an inch each day.
- An average total of one pound of hair will be removed by daily shaving over a period of sixteen years.
- You will spend close to 3,350 hours shaving if you live an average lifetime.
- If you never shaved, you'd have a built-in mop in a beard nearly thirty feet long.

Question: You mentioned taking a shower after washing the face and right before shaving. I have a long commute to my office on public transportation, and I'm afraid I'll miss the train. Anything wrong with showering at night?

Answer: No. Just be sure to allow time to let your beard soak before shaving.

Remember that a dry whisker is as tough as a copper wire of the same thickness. The real secret of good shaving is getting that tough bit of hair—and all its companions—as un-dry as possible. Water—even more than shaving cream—is the thing that makes those whiskers soft enough to cut. Without it, you'd ruin your razor blade in a matter of seconds and end up looking like you'd been in a fight with an alley cat. That is why I suggested a preferred order of things for your morning grooming ritual.

The shower, after your regular face scrubbing, will give you another opportunity to get plenty of water on your beard. It's preferable to not use hot water directly on your face, but the warmer water of the shower will also provide a bit of steam that will help soften the beard. You will have removed the excess oil from your face with the wash and exfoliation, and that will make it easier for the facial hair to soak up water. Whiskers, happily, are thirsty little devils that can expand in volume by a full third in two minutes by soaking up water. That means you and your razor will only have to do two-thirds of the work in cutting them down to size.

Rule: You can't overuse water before shaving. Allow two minutes for whiskers to soak.

Have you had the experience of shaving before work only to find that your beard feels like sandpaper by the end of lunch? If so, it doesn't necessarily mean that you're doing it wrong or that you have a dull blade. Studies have shown that the average beard grows most between the hours of 8:00 A.M. and 1:00 P.M. In the same vein, scientific studies indicate that the beard seems to grow more during warm seasons, periods of unusual stress and fatigue, and bouts of heavy drinking.

Question: If water does most of the softening, why do we need to use any kind of shaving cream?

Shaving cream serves two important functions: (1) a proper shaving cream will lock the moisture in the hair follicles and delay the process of evaporation, and (2) a good cream will act as an effective lubricant that reduces the drag on your razor as you pull it through the stubble and down your face. Also, the better shaving creams tend to keep the whiskers more upright if they are applied to the shaving area against the natural grain of hair growth.

Question: I'll buy your advice about washing in lukewarm water, but are you sure hot water isn't better for shaving?

Answer: To paraphrase Gertrude Stein, "A whisker is a whisker is a whisker. And water is water is water."

Water is essential for comfortable close shaving because the whiskers are highly absorbent. Once the area to be shaved is cleaned of excess oil, it doesn't really matter if the water is hot or cold. The individual hairs will greedily suck it up. The only possible advantage of using very hot water is that it may soak its way into the whisker a bit faster. But are those few seconds of time worth the risk of what the hot water can do to the skin from which those whiskers grow? My answer to that is an emphatic *no*.

It is tough to break habits of long standing, and I know that men have been using hot water for shaving for a long time. But it really serves very little purpose of a constructive nature, and continued use can harm the overall structure of your face. Try shaving in the manner I have suggested, using lukewarm water. I think you'll be both surprised and pleased with the results.

If you want to use hot water, use it on the blade of your razor. Very hot water will clean the blade better and actually make it perform somewhat better as you shave.

> *Question*: I've been using a good aerosol shaving cream
> for years, and I like it. It's more convenient and
> less messy.

There's no doubt that spraying on a thick coating of foam is much more convenient than fiddling around with the old mug of shaving soap and a brush. On the other hand, sticking the foil-wrapped tray of a frozen TV dinner in the oven is easier than preparing a real home-cooked meal or getting duded up to go out to a posh restaurant. But which tastes better and is better for you?

I made brief mention earlier that aerosol shaving products are mostly a combination of water and propellant, up to 90 percent. It stands to reason that they are going to provide less protection for the skin against the abrasiveness of the razor blade. If you've been using an aerosol for a long time with fairly good results, it's unlikely that you are allergic to the propellant, but many men are. Some of the additives in aerosol foams—particularly lime and lemon scents—can cause phototoxic reactions in the form of bad sunburns or rashes on men who are sensitive to strong sunlight. Finally, aerosol foams are the worst buy, giving you the fewest shaves for the dollar.

Recommended Shaving Aids
(In Order of Preference)

1. Shaving cream
2. Shaving gel

3. Shaving soap
4. Shaving foam

All About Shaving Creams

It's important to remember that the beard area of a man's face is always the driest portion of the epidermis, regardless of individual skin type. Even men with excessively oily skin will usually have that problem only on the chin, a part of the T zone. So, generally speaking, we want to avoid shaving preparations that might add to the drying.

Because the two main functions of a shaving cream are to form a block that will retain the water in whiskers and to lubricate the path of the razor, the fewer additives in your shave cream the better. Shaving means that you are literally scraping the skin with a sharp instrument, and this is an abrasive task, no matter how expertly you perform it. The hydrocarbons of aerosol foams, the citric acids, menthols, and even the scents of the products are likely to leave your skin feeling more rather than less irritated.

As in the case of good face soap, I would prefer not to get into a listing of specific name brands. Because shaving is something every male has to do, manufacturers have been very energetic in producing a wide variety of products that have been seriously tested and are available in supermarkets, drug stores, and department stores. Again, you can pay as much as you like, but there is little advantage in selecting an expensive designer-name product.

I have added shaving soap to my list of preferred products specifically for men who have problems with very oily skin, even in the shaving area. Shaving soap has a tendency toward drying and should not be used for men of other skin types. Any of the reasonably priced mug soaps would be acceptable for oily-skinned men, on a starting basis, as would one of the lathering shave creams that come in a tube.

I want to emphasize again that I am not shilling for any product manufacturer, and I know how comfortable we can become with an old habit. However, in the interest of a workable skin care program, you would be taking a giant stride forward by throwing away the

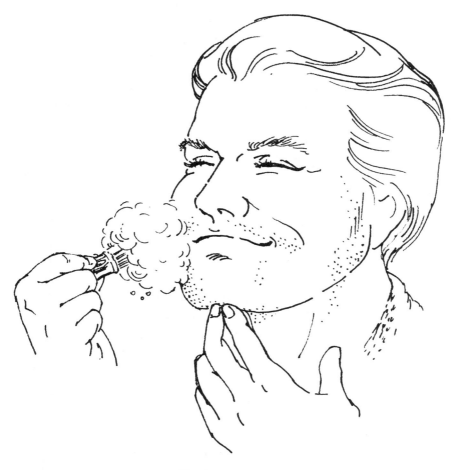

Shaving cream

can of aerosol foam and investing in a good shaving cream that comes in a tube. If you are hung up on aerosols, switch to a gel. Gels are thicker, can be easily spread over the shaving area with your fingertips, and provide much better lubrication to ease the way of the razor's cutting edge.

Brushless shaving creams, which are packaged in handy tubes, are your best bet for getting a close shave that will be free of irritation and do no damage to your skin. The pH factor of these creams is very low, making them gentle on even the driest skin, and they contain emulsifiers to keep the water and oil ingredients from separating, lubricants to reduce friction, and humectants to seal the water into the whiskers. If you have already cleaned and washed your face according to my suggestions, these creams will give you a fine shave.

There are many fine creams on the market in a variety of price ranges. Strangely, some of the higher-priced creams made by so-called designer companies contain a preservative called paraben that could cause an allergic reaction in men with ultra-sensitive skin. Perfectly good brushless shave creams are produced by such familiar names as Gillette, Mennen, Barbasol, and Noxema. These creams contain a variety of natural ingredients—olive oil, peanut oil, lanolin, etc.—that will make shaving easier. It should be remembered that brushless shave creams are not designed to provide copious amounts of lather. They do the job without it.

Shaving Shortcuts

1. All men past the age range of thirty-five to forty should always use a good brushless shave cream. It will lessen drying.
2. Young men with excessively oily skin might try lathering the beard before showering as an easy way to promote drying.

Choose Your Weapon

Considering the endless variety of shaving instruments on the market today, it's a bit surprising that earlier in this century nearly all men were slicing off their whiskers with the favorite scalpel of Sweeney Todd, the demon barber of Fleet Street. The dangerous straight razor was actually the favorite tool of most Americans until the doughboys of World War I were issued double-edged safety razors with the proviso that they shave every day.

Today, it's usually only the barber who has the nerve to wield a straight razor. At home we have an option of double-edged, single-edged, adjustable, twin-blade, pivoting twin-blade, triple-blade, ejectors, cutting bands, throw-away plastics, and several types of electric razors. I believe that a wet shave with a good cream is more beneficial for the face. Otherwise, I don't think the selection of a razor is that important. After all, it's the blade that really counts.

With that in mind, there is much to be said for the twin-blade razors that were first introduced in the early 1970s. The theory of twin-blade shaving is sound. The razor blade actually pulls the whisker out of its follicle pocket while it is being cut. The second blade is designed to nip off that portion of the hair left standing before it retracts back into the follicle pocket, giving a closer, smoother shave. Twin-blade razors, both rigid and pivoting, have won wide acceptance and are designed and promoted now by several companies. Personally, I find it annoying that whisker debris and shaving cream tend to collect between the blades, getting in the way of a really good shave. Of course, this can be minimized by repeated rinsings with hot water during the course of your shave.

> *Rule*: No matter what safety razor you use, rinse the blade often with hot water before, during, and after the shave.

In today's terminology, the razor is the instrument that holds the blade which does the actual cutting of the whiskers. The technology of blade manufacturers has advanced to the point that the least expensive blades—costing fifteen cents or less—will do a good job of shaving if they are not used too long. Better to invest a few cents more and buy a coated blade that will ease the pull on the whiskers and also keep its edge better. The better blades are coated with platinum and Teflon to reduce drag. They're well worth the extra money.

If you find that you often nick yourself while shaving, especially after you have begun this skin care program, it would be very worthwhile to consider changing your razor and blades. In selecting a razor, pick one that literally feels right for you, both in your hand and on your face. Shaving cuts are almost always the result of an attempt to hurry, a cumbersome razor, too much pressure, or a dull blade.

> *Rule*: Set a regular schedule for changing blades. It's easy to forget to change, and a dull blade can bulldoze your skin care program.

Knowing the Territory

A good, safe shave cream, a comfortable razor, a sharp, coated blade—what's left? It's time to reconnoiter the area about to be attacked. *Renovated* is perhaps a more appropriate word. Nevertheless, it's wise to gather intelligence about the opponent. Just as skin color seems to dictate beard density (white men have generally thicker beards, black men somewhat less dense, oriental men the sparsest facial hair), whiskers generally concentrate heavily toward the center of the face on all men. The thickest growth is found on the chin and above the upper lip.

The beard is not only denser on the chin and above the upper lip, but the individual whiskers are also coarser in these areas. That means the more time we give them to soak up water, the easier they'll be to cut. By the same token, these areas could use a thicker coating of cream to retain the moisture in the hair. They should be shaved last.

Shaving Order

1. Jawline beneath the sideburns
2. Cheeks
3. Neck
4. Mustache area
5. Chin

Another reminder: you can get a closer shave by working against the grain, in the opposite direction from which the whiskers naturally grow. I consider this practice, like too much blade pressure, counterproductive to good skin care. Shaving this way will result in needlessly stretching the skin and will also result in needless cuts and the possibility of ingrown hairs. You'd be better off shaving twice a day or simply changing to a sharp new blade more often. When completing your shave, remember to rinse very thoroughly. It wouldn't hurt to spend a couple of minutes making certain that all the shaving cream residue is off your face. We don't want to negate the benefits of the careful skin cleaning we did before the shave.

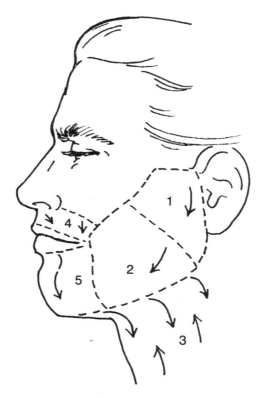

Shaving order

Question: I'm disturbed by your suggestion that I not use an after-shave lotion. I've got an expensive favorite that I've been using, and the women are wild about it. It's become part of my masculine identity because it's an acceptable scent. Even my dad thought it was okay to use after shave.

My opposition to after shaves has nothing to do with scent. You can take too much alcohol for your own good *internally*, and too much alcohol applied to the skin *externally* can be nearly as destructive. Alcohol is one of the world's best drying agents, and nearly all after-shave products have alcohol as the main ingredient. Men with dry, dehydrated, or aging skin might be better off selecting some unenlightened person they dislike and making him a present of the after shave now in the bathroom cabinet.

If you have normal, combination, or oily skin, you can get away with a very light splash of after shave for the time being. But steady use of such an astringent is going to get to you eventually. Alcohol-based products certainly are good for removing excess oil from the skin, and they do suffice to make the pores smaller on a very temporary basis. But even men with ultra-oily skin will get no lasting benefits from its steady use. The sebaceous glands will only work harder to replace the oil that has been eliminated. So it's a no-win situation for everyone. I strongly suggest that everyone use the procedure I outlined earlier: (1) After rinsing and drying, coat the shaved area with a fine spray of mineral water. (2) Apply a thin coat of commercial, water-based moisturizer to the beard area. (3) For a pleasant scent, put a tiny dab of men's cologne or after shave on the jawline close to the ear.

This simple and, up to now, unorthodox after-shave routine will leave you feeling refreshed, smelling good, and looking much better in the years ahead.

Let's say you have a bottle of expensive after-shave lotion, and you can't bear to part with it. You also have a very oily T zone. Don't use the after shave on the dry beard area. Use spare amounts of the lotion on the most oily parts of the T zone.

Electric Shaving: The Pros and Cons

Question: I notice you haven't talked about shaving with an electric razor. I use one, and I think it's the greatest—easier and faster. How about that?

Answer: I haven't discussed electric shaving yet because, in the interest of skin care, getting there "fustest" doesn't always leave you with the "mostest"!

Here's to the manufacturers of electric razors! By and large, those companies have done a fine job of easing the drudgery of daily shaving, particularly when you consider how much they have improved their product over a relatively short period of time. Most electric razors can give you a pretty close shave in a process that is less messy and certainly faster. However, I'm going to withhold some of my praise until they perfect a system that will allow you to use an electric razor with water and shaving cream.

In almost all cases, a wet shave is more beneficial to the skin than a dry shave. That is precisely why I went into great detail about the best method of shaving in the preceding paragraphs. A good wet shave will not only do an excellent job of cutting off the whiskers, but it will also benefit the skin when accompanied by all the before, during, and after preparations I have suggested. Unfortunately, to a large extent dry shaving will only cut off the whiskers.

To be more exact, electric shaving will shear the whiskers. In essence, an electric razor is a shearing machine, a refined version of the electric clippers that a military barber uses to give a new recruit the traditional skinhead haircut. I don't mean to simply dismiss electric razors as worthless. They can be a valuable tool when used in conjunction with your wet shaving program. But I would advise using them as a supplementary aid rather than your main shaving instrument.

Just consider what was said earlier about the nature of the strand of facial hair known as a whisker: it soaks up water like the proverbial camel, and it cuts much easier when water-logged. You don't have that advantage when using an electric razor, whether it's a rotary, a foil head, or a slot head razor. Each of those will simply whirr its way through the hair on your face, often leaving the whiskers with jagged edges as they are tugged and chopped away from your skin. Remember, too, that water and a good shave cream cause the individual hairs to stand more erect, enabling you to cut them away with less drag. You don't have that advantage with electric shaving.

Question: What about using an electric preshave?

Now we're right back to the controversy about using a regular after-shave lotion. Like after-shave preparations, preshave lotions are largely alcohol. You pretty well have to use a preshave before using an electric razor because the normal oil and moisture on the face will make it nearly impossible for the electric razor to mow down the dry whiskers. In doing so, you are deliberately drying your skin before you start your shave. The companies that produce men's grooming products are aware of this situation, and for men with dry skin they also produce a product for use as a preshave that is meant to soak up the facial oil rather than strip it away.

Preshave talcs, as these products are called, are composed mainly of talcum powder and are less drying and harmful to already dry, aging, or dehydrated skin. But after using this product, the electric-shaver user is still faced with the problem of scrubbing the powder away to keep it from clogging the pores. In the final analysis, doing everything as recommended, do you still believe that electric shaving is easier and faster? I'm not so sure.

If you already own a good electric razor that gives you good results, I certainly don't suggest that you get rid of it. If you have normal or healthy combination skin, you can safely continue to use it at those times when you are in an inordinate hurry to get somewhere. The same can be said for those with minor cases of dry skin. I do not think it advisable for men with aging or dehydrated skin to use an electric razor except on rare occasions. In the long run, purposeful wet shaving is better for all skin types, at least until they perfect a system of wet shaving with an electric razor.

Electric Razor Shortcuts

1. An electric razor can be helpful for quick touch-ups.
2. An electric razor with a trimmer attachment can be an invaluable tool for keeping a mustache or a full or partial beard looking its neatest.

Problems, Problems, Problems

Question: I'm one of those guys who suffers from terminal five o'clock shadow. What can I do about it? After dark I look like the Werewolf of London.

The so-called five o'clock shadow problem has plagued millions of men for a long time. There's really no easy way around it. You shave in the morning in order to look good for the job and discover that you look like a candidate for Skid Row when it's time to go home or head out for a bit of fun. The first thing you should understand is that you have no special skin or whisker problem. Your beard probably isn't even heavier. It's only darker.

Here's another area where we can learn a lesson from those

gorgeous people who have no need to shave their faces. How many women do you know who would even dream of going out in the evening without fussing over their makeup and hair? We men don't have to endure that cosmetic nonsense, but a second light shave should be considered the masculine counterpart. If you're going out on the town with your wife, you'll have time for a relaxing wet shave while she's making her preparations. If you're going on an important date, business or social, soon after work, you've found the perfect opportunity to use that electric razor that you've largely abandoned in favor of regular shaving. An electric shaver that you can use in the car or on the plane is the perfect instrument to have handy in your briefcase or the drawer of your office desk. I would caution against overdoing it, but an electric razor or a second regular shave are the only alternatives for men who worry about a persistent five o'clock shadow.

> *Question*: I'm over twenty-one, but I still get big zits from time to time which I assume are a carryover from the acne I had as a tennager. What's the scoop on shaving with a condition like this?

I'll be making specific suggestions on how to deal with acne later in this book, but I would first advise you to see a medical doctor if the problem is severe. That same advice holds if you also have a problem with warts or moles in the beard area. As far as an occasional problem with a pimple, go ahead with the regular wet shaving routine that I have suggested, taking care that you don't slice through the blemish. Again, a good soaking of the whiskers in tepid water and a thick coat of shaving cream will do the job. Make certain to shave with the natural grain of the beard. Shaving against the grain will produce further irritation. Also avoid using an electric razor, which can induce permanent scarring if you mow through an acne eruption.

> *Question*: No matter what kind of razor I use, I seem to end up with my face very irritated, almost like a rash. What could be causing it?

The most likely villain in your scenario is the excess force you apply to make up for the dullness of your blade. If you are giving your whiskers a proper soaking with tepid water and keeping the moisture locked in and the whiskers lubricated with a good heavy shave cream, it's probably the blade-pressure ratio that's causing the problem. If you shave with an electric razor, the same difficulty can arise. Men with sensitive skin should limit or eliminate electric shaving. If you're innocent of all these possible errors, it's time to check the support substances you use for shaving. If you are using a soap or shave cream too strong for your skin, you can go to the nearest drug store and buy a package of Squibb Nitrazine papers. Rub a bit of your soap or shave cream on one of the papers, and a color chart will explain its degree of alkalinity or acidity. You may need milder products, but make sure you are handling the physical end of shaving correctly before bothering with tests.

> *Question*: I have a problem that's driving me bananas, and I can't seem to get rid of it. I'm talking about ingrown hairs. Is there any simple way to keep them from happening?

The greatest weapon ever invented for the control of ingrown hairs is an instrument that has fallen out of favor a bit in recent years: the adjustable razor. Ingrown hairs are always caused by improper shaving, and they are especially prevalent among men who have naturally curly hair. They can occur anywhere in the beard area, but especially on the neck where so many men are inclined to shave against the grain.

Doctors even have a Latin name for ingrown hairs and their resultant shaving bumps—*pseudofolliculitis barbae*—but all it amounts to is the tendency of a jagged-edged curly whisker to bend and reattach itself into the skin under the pressure of shaving. These things can become painfully annoying, so much so that some men resort to wax depilatories and even electrolysis in their eagerness to get rid of them. The easiest cure is to simply stop shaving, but not many of us can afford that luxury. You'll be on your way to a cure if you abandon shaving with an electric razor and also swear to stop using excessive force and working against the grain when you use a blade razor.

Adjustable razors are still being sold, although you may have to look around a bit to find one. They are the metal safety razors that have a movable gizmo in the handle, or the plastic numbers that have a lever near the blade, which allows you to dial the closeness of your shave. Continue your normal wet shave routine, but set the blade adjustment to the point farthest from your skin when you work the areas where you have ingrown-hair problems. I think you'll notice less discomfort from the very beginning, but the process will take a bit of time. As the pain eases, adjust the blade a notch closer to the skin in each succeeding week. By the end of a month, or sooner, the difficulty should be corrected.

> *Question*: I know you think a dull razor and too much pressure cause cuts, but what about a sharp one? Every time I insert a new blade, I get all kinds of nicks. I've tried the old stick-pieces-of-toilet-paper-on-the-cut routine. I look like I have albino measles, and it doesn't work. How do you stop bleeding?

To answer the first question, a fresh blade requires even less pressure than one you've used a couple of times. You should change blades often to avoid using undue pressure, and once you're accustomed to that routine you'll be even more careful. The toilet-paper routine falls under the heading of another Old Dad's tale. It's easier to invest a few pieces of change in a device that's been on the market for years: a styptic pencil. It's available at all drug stores, comes in liquid or stick form, and does a great job on minor bleeding.

Safe Shaving—Quick Menu

1. The wet shave is preferred for all skin types on a regular basis.
2. Shave after cleaning the face and showering.
3. Men with extra oily skin may want to apply shaving soap before entering the shower.
4. A thick brushless shaving cream is best for most skin types.
5. Allow lukewarm water two minutes to soak into whiskers, and then apply shave cream.
6. Use a razor that feels comfortable in your hand and on your face.
7. Coated—especially Teflon or platinum—blades give a smoother and closer shave.
8. Always shave with the grain, in the direction of natural beard growth.

9. Avoid undue pressure with the blade.

10. Shave jawline, cheeks, and neck first, upper lip and chin last.

11. Rinse the blade before, during, and after the shave with hot water.

12. Rinse face with great care to remove all traces of shave cream, and pat dry.

13. Avoid standard after-shave lotions which are mainly alcohol and too drying on the skin.

14. Use regular after-shave lotion as an astringent on overly oily T zone, or put a dab near each ear for scent.

15. Spray fine water mist on shaved area and cover with disappearing water-based men's moisturizer.

16. Use electric razor primarily for emergency touch-ups or extra shaves to dispel five o'clock shadow.

17. Use an adjustable razor set at maximum distance to correct problem of ingrown hairs.

5

The Sportsman's Skin: Toning Face and Body

Don't let this chapter title fool you. It's for you even if you see yourself as a ninety-seven-pound weakling whose biggest physical test is hoisting a stein of beer. Sports and the workplace, particularly outdoors, create problems for many men that are distinctly different from those experienced by women. Martina Navratilova, Greta Waitz, and Nancy Lopez not excepted, men have been conditioned to use their larger muscles more strenuously whether they're engaged in a one-on-one game of basketball on a city playground or dashing down a long airport corridor to grab a plane.

Strenuous excerise with proper precautions is excellent for the skin. Your skin is a body organ; therefore, it benefits from a regular routine of exercise just like almost all the other organs of your body. With the fitness craze of recent years, you are already familiar with the overall advantages of a good exercise program. Body exercise is good for your mental and physical health. We can see and feel the beneficial results of exercise on our bodies and major internal organs, but that same kind of exercise can also be of great value to your skin—the skin of your body and face.

Exercise helps the face by:

1. Enhancing blood circulation
2. Supplying more oxygen for the skin
3. Stimulating the sweat glands
4. Encouraging us to concentrate on skin tone

However, the strenuous kinds of exercises that most of us engage in can bring on special problems because of the exertion required to perform them. A similar situation exists among men who work at jobs that require physical strength or dexterity, particularly if they perform those tasks out-of-doors. In both instances, I'm talking specifically about possible harm to the skin of the face. Again, since our bodies are usually clothed, their youthful condition is not nearly as instantly apparent or important as our faces. In this chapter you'll learn ways to protect and preserve your face while you build your body.

If You Do It Outdoors, Be Careful

Men spend much more time outside in pursuit of their livelihoods or leisure sports, and that is the main reason why we have facial skin that's a bit thicker than the average woman's. Unfortunately, that affords us only a tiny bit more protection. When you consider that many women wear makeup of some kind, their skin is actually less vulnerable to possible harm from weather and environmental pollution than ours. And that's the bare-faced truth. If you are seriously interested in keeping your face as youthful and good-looking as possible, it's important to be aware of the dangers you face each time you go out the front door.

Old Sol Is No Pal

The ultraviolet rays of the sun will do more to determine the kind of facial skin you're going to be carrying into your middle years than any other factor except normal aging and heredity. If your favorite sport is played in the great outdoors, your face is susceptible to the sun's damaging rays, in summer and in winter. For that matter, if your job keeps you outside a good deal of the time, you should also be aware of the problems the sun can cause you. And we're not talking about the unsightliness of a peeling sunburn but about serious long-term skin damage.

Question: It's pretty hard to get away from the sun. Am I supposed to wear one of those plastic bubble suits or live in a dark cave?

Answer: I wish the choices were that simple. Unfortunately, the relationship you establish with the sun is one of those so-called life choices, a matter of instant gratification or long-term success.

Obviously, nobody can stay out of the sun at all times, and we'd all be in bad shape if the sun decided to take a permanent vacation. But it's extremely important from the viewpoint of good skin care that we understand that it's dangerous to become too buddy-buddy with the sun. It's the enormous energy of the sun that causes everything on our planet to grow, but let those waving fields of grain go without moisture for a time and they will become acres of stunted, twisted vegetable debris. The same sun that keeps growing things alive can also kill. The skin of every human being, male or female, will suffer the same fate without proper protection.

Remember the three main skin layers, the epidermis, dermis, and hypodermis? Those unseen but omnipotent ultraviolet rays of the sun can wreak havoc with all three layers of the skin on your face. Both the first sunburn of the year and the ultimate tan are the result of the sun baking your epidermis. As we know, that epidermis is composed of dead cells in any event so relatively little damage is done here. It's under the epidermis that the sun takes great glee in its seek and destroy mission in a manner that makes Rambo look like a world-class wimp. The worst part of this story is that we're not even aware of this damage until after it's done. Our faces may smart and burn from a bad sunburn, but that will go away as the epidermis cools and peels. However, while it's been burning the epidermis, the ultraviolet has also been baking the dermis and hypodermis, literally frying the collagen, the fatty tissue, and the elastin network that gives your skin elasticity and your face its form.

This is the ultimate danger in being a sun worshipper. In most men, the sun is the number one cause of premature aging of the skin. The sun was Mother Nature's clothes dryer long before someone invented the electric type. It is also the best possible skin dryer. If the sun was capable of baking bricks for the Pueblo Indians, just think what it's doing to your layers of skin. Again, the real devastation is taking place under the epidermis and causing damage that cannot really be repaired. Regular overexposure to solar radiation is going to give you an outer skin layer that will become thick, tough, and lined with knots of cross-linked tissue. Your epidermis will become badly wrinkled before its time, and your collagen will become badly depleted, and that can lead to middle-aged facial folds that only a plastic surgeon can make better.

Question: Is it true that too much sunbathing can lead to skin cancer?

Cancer experts have already proved that overexposure to the sun is not only a contributing factor in skin cancer but its number one cause. In fact, most medical doctors would prefer that you avoid the sun like the plague. It's no coincidence that there are more cases of skin cancer in the southern portions of the United States, where the sun is hotter, than in the north. Fortunately, most skin cancers are curable and pose no very serious problems other than the discomfort and expense necessary to remove them. But the fact that the sun has the power to create that kind of problem is evidence of the less immediately noticeable damage it is doing to your skin.

Question: I think tans look great on other people, but I can't seem to get one. I only burn. Why is that?

The ability to tan has everything to do with ethnic background. I'd be willing to bet that your ancestors came from somewhere in northern Europe. People of Celtic, Scandinavian, German, Anglo-Saxon, and other origins of northern Europe are fair-skinned and more likely to burn before they'll tan. This is not always the case, but these people usually do not tan as well as their friends whose forebears came from southern Europe, the Middle East, or anyplace close to the Mediterranean.

I didn't go into the matter of melanin when we examined the makeup of the skin earlier. This is a good time to do so. Melanin ranks right up with land-grabbing and religious differences as the biggest causes of trouble in the world because it is the substance that determines the hue, shade, and color of human skin. But when it comes to our relationship with the sun, melanin is the good guy. It's the only natural protection we have against Old Sol's harmful rays. Melanin is simply pigment cells that are located at the very bottom of the epidermis. They are there specifically to protect the dermis from harmful ultraviolet rays. In the wonderful natural order of things, humans living closest to the sun's rays—at the equator—were provided with more melanin and darker skins. The farther from the equator, the less melanin and the lighter the skin. Generally speaking, the darker the skin, the fewer problems you'll have from the sun. However, nobody is completely safe from ultraviolet sun rays.

> *Question*: You've got me totally confused. I happen to think that everybody looks better with a nice tan. Go to any beach and it's obvious that my thought isn't original. Is the whole world nuts except you?
>
> *Answer*: In the past, we suffered foolish pain and strife in our society because of the wide variety of skin colors among our citizens. Some lighter people considered the darker ones inferior. Nevertheless, hordes of the same lighter-skinned folk were flocking to beaches to get darker, while some of those with more melanin bought bleaching cream, hoping to become lighter. Does this answer your question?

"To tan or not to tan?" is a question worthy of Hamlet. I know that asking a healthy young male to give up a summer on the beach is tantamount to suggesting that he forget about sex. So I'm not going to do that. But I cannot stress too strongly the danger you run in spending too much time on the inviting sands or other areas that can be just as hazardous to the health of your skin. It's ironic that a good tan is very much a status symbol today, because that is a complete reversal of the thinking of just a few decades ago.

The epithet *redneck* is still in vogue to describe someone who is uneducated, prejudiced, and otherwise can't distinguish between his aft and his elbow. But examine the composition of the word. Its literal meaning is someone with a red neck, a man who has to work outside at some stoop labor that causes his neck to become badly sunburned. It grew out of the old white-collar–blue-collar class struggle. Someone who had to labor for a living simply was not quite good enough. Sunburns and suntans were to be avoided at all costs. Today, we've come almost full circle. Most of us feel self-conscious if we show up at beach or pool looking like an unbaked bagel.

Question: So how did things get turned around? Who started the tanning craze?

To say that one sickness bred another would probably be the shortest and most accurate answer to the question. In the 1920s, doctors discovered that ample amounts of sunshine in clean-air places like Arizona helped the healing process of those who had contracted tuberculosis. Those wealthy enough to take such sabbaticals impressed their healthy friends with their remarkably fit looks, and the tanning fad began to gather followers among "the beautiful people." Before long, the fact that you were tan came to mean that you had leisure time. You weren't required to spend your day toiling at some menial job in a dark and dreary factory. There's no doubt that the shrinking size of women's bathing suits has done nothing to impede the steady flow of rampant males to beach and pool.

Question: I have very oily skin. Wouldn't the sun help me dry it?

Right you are! Here's another case where men with oily skin have a built-in advantage over the rest of us, particularly if the oily skin accompanies a somewhat darker complexion. Taken in sensible doses, sunlight can be very helpful in getting the face back to normal. Generally speaking, it's dark-complexioned men with somewhat oily skin who tan best and look best with the tan. Just remember, even dark-complexioned black men can suffer burns and skin damage from too much time in the sun. In any event, continue your regular skin care program with extra effort placed on exfoliating the dead cells to avoid clogged pores.

Question: I'm too restless to be a beach freak, but I do love sailing in the summer and skiing in the winter. Any special precautions needed here?

Special precautions are advisable in any sport that requires you to spend lengthy time in the bright sun. Remember, the harmful ultraviolet rays can cause trouble even on overcast days when the sun doesn't seem bright. That's easy to forget. Lying on a beach or at poolside is the most dangerous because you're wearing a minimum of clothing and catching ultraviolet over almost all of your anatomy. Your face—our primary concern—remains uncovered no matter what the sport. Your favorites, sailing and skiing, are two of the most dangerous for proper skin maintenance because they take place on water and snow, which rank with sand as the greatest reflectors of the sun's ultraviolet shrinkers. Both sports also leave you open to a good case of windburn which can be nearly as bad for your face as sunburn. Skiing can be particularly rough on your skin because it takes place at a time when many don't expect to be burned. However, the higher altitude means less atmosphere to block out the ultraviolet rays, and the snow acts as a reflector to blast your face with sunlight.

> *Question*: Look, I have pretty fair skin, and I always burn in the beginning before it changes into a tan. That's part of the natural process. right?

Wrong! Burning and tanning are separate processes that are vaguely related. Burning is exactly what the term implies. The sun's rays literally burn the topmost layers of skin as surely as if you had climbed into a hot oven. Most people, especially the fair-skinned, consider this normal and the only way they can get a tan. Even men with darker complexions turn red before tanning at the beginning of the season. But their redness soon disappears as the melanin rises to the surface and become a deep tan. Burning does not lead to tanning, because the burned skin will peel away and the ultraviolet reaction will cause the burning process to start all over again the next time the victim goes into the sun.

> *Question*: It sounds so hopeless. Isn't there any way a fair-skinned guy can get a decent tan?

In some very fair-skinned, blue-eyed men it is virtually hopeless. Continued overexposure to the sun is potentially disastrous and, in the opinion of most dermatologists, not really worth the time and effort. Assuming you have some supply of normal melanin and a great deal of patience and determination, it's possible for you to get a light bronzing eventually. However, if you have dry, dehydrated, or aging skin, it would be best if you avoided the sun. Remember, long-term baking is sure to leave you with a face that only your mother could love.

Question: I don't have particularly light skin, but sometimes I get very painful sunburns and also some kind of rash. Any idea what my problem might be?

It sounds like you may be a victim of photosensitization. In other words, your skin has become unusually sensitive to the sun's rays because of something you have taken internally or applied externally. A good dermatologist can quickly pinpoint your problem. Many substances cause this kind of reaction in people: citric oils and juices in after-shave lotions, deodorant soaps, and even certain prescription drugs. If sunning brings on a painful burn or rash that is not normal for you, best check with a doctor.

Rule: Nobody, regardless of skin type, should plan a long session under the hot sun without proper before, during, and after protection.

There's no argument that by today's standards nearly every man looks younger and more fit with a good tan. There's also no doubt that most of us would have youthful-looking skin later in life if we didn't become compulsive about soaking up those rays. How about a sensible compromise? Starting from nothing in the late 1920s, the suntan lotion industry now takes in close to $100 million per year. In the beginning, tanning products were little more than simple oils that enabled the skin to fry rather than bake. Fortunately, with good research that revealed how damaging overexposure to the sun could be to human skin, the tanning industry has come up with a wide variety of products that enables almost all of us to pursue our active outdoor interests without calamitous effect. Using the best of these products—and a good dollop of common sense—will enable you to enjoy your season in the sun without regrets.

As in the case of other commercial products, I am not going to recommend any specific brand name. There are numerous effective tanning safeguards on the market. I will recommend that you use a sunscreen rather than a simple lotion. I also advise that you buy one that contains para-aminobenzoic acid, which will probably be abbreviated on the label as PABA. Exhaustive tests have shown that this is the best agent for preventing premature aging and skin cancer from exposure to the sun. Sunscreens have been designed to give you the amount of protection you need for your skin type. They are numbered to identify the product's "sun protection factor," usually from 1 to 15. Those who burn easiest should stick to the higher numbers while those who rarely burn can utilize the numbers at the lower end of the scale. Such products, chosen in accordance to your skin type, will allow you to spend considerably more time in the sun without harmful effect than you could with no skin protection.

Sensible Sunning

1. Everyone burns sooner under a tropical sun.
2. Everyone burns sooner at high altitude, summer or winter.
3. Don't attempt to rush a tan; build it slowly.
4. The lighter your skin, the less sun you can afford.
5. Everyone should use a suitable sunscreen on his first exposure of the season.
6. Keep the midday sun—between 10:00 A.M. and 2:00 P.M.— the exclusive reserve of Noel Coward, mad dogs, and Englishmen.
7. Fair-skinned men should always use a suitable sunscreen.
8. Anyone who must spend long hours in the sun—lifeguards, golf or tennis pros, any outdoor worker—should always wear an appropriate sunscreen, regardless of skin type.
9. Men with excessively dry, dehydrated, or aging skin must either avoid the sun or use a sun block product that will effectively nullify the harmful sun rays.
10. Watch out for photosensitization caused by a substance either in or on your person.

We're right back where we started. However, forewarned is forearmed. Once you know the dangers of overdoing your time in the sun and the sensible approach that will allow you to have your cake and eat it too, the rest is squarely up to you. This has been a lengthy warning, but it cannot be emphasized too strongly. There's nothing so macho or appealing about being a bronzed warrior in your youth and discovering that you have a face with all the leathery glamour of a floppy old ski boot when you celebrate your thirty-eighth birthday. Without proper precaution, your friend the sun will do that to you.

> *Question*: Almost all of my outdoor recreation time is spent on golf, and I think I may have another problem with the sun. I can't stand bright sunshine when I'm playing, and I do a lot of squinting which probably causes all the little wrinkles around my eyes. Are blue eyes extra sensitive to the sun?

The latest studies show there's a good chance that this is the case. You probably have a fairly light complexion to go with your blue eyes, and the sun on the golf course is probably drying your skin at the same time as it's causing you to squint. You should apply some medium-range sunscreen before you tee off. You'd also be wiser to wear a visored golf cap. Strong sun is also harmful to your hair. Fortunately, the people who make sunglasses have also come up with improvements that keep them from flying off when you launch a long drive. The same ultraviolet rays that are harmful to skin, coupled with infrared rays, can give fits to your eyes when you're working or playing in the sun. Manufacturers of sunglasses have now perfected a variety of lenses that are both practical and good-looking. They come in a number of frames that are shaped to enhance the configuration of the face and avoid annoying slipping down the nose. Men whose sports or work keeps them in bright sunlight—fishermen, sailors, lifeguards, policemen—might benefit from constant density lenses. Other sportsmen—golfers, tennis players—might prefer photochromic lenses which automatically adjust to the intensity of the sun. Squinting because of sun glare and laughing are the chief causes of the so-called crow's feet around the eyes. Everyone's skin is drier and thinner around the eyes, so a good pair of sunglasses should be considered a worthy investment.

> *Question*: I belong to a health club that has one of those tanning machines. What's the scoop on those?

Basically, the rule is simple: regard that man-made brightness with the same respect you give the sun. Artificial tanning in health clubs and in special salons has become a booming industry in recent years. Fortunately, the tanning machines in health clubs have printed instructions that clearly warn you about the possible dangers. The owners of salons that specialize in artificial tanning, for their own protection as well as yours, are careful that you don't suffer from overexposure. If you normally tan easily, they can give you a relatively harmless glow even in midwinter. As usual, men with fair, dry, dehydrated, or aging skin should approach such devices with caution.

> *Question*: What do you think about bronzers that you apply to your face?

They're basically harmless but also not terribly satisfactory for a lot of men. The dihydroxy acetone in most of these products simply dyes your skin a color that looks a bit like a tan. Problems arise because the color comes out more orange than tan on some men. If you get some of that cream on your hair or clothing, they also take on a warm orange glow. Because the substance actually dyes the upper cell layers of the epidermis, it's important to apply it smoothly to avoid a blotchy, uneven look. Taken with a bit of natural sunlight or a tanning light, it tends to look more real. But don't forget that a bronzer tan is not real and will offer you no protection against sunburn.

> *Question*: I'm a guy who always burns and never tans. I read an ad about a pill that tans you. What do you think?

I think it would work better for you than the sun. A number of pills or capsules have been devised recently that promise to give you something that can pass as a tan without the destructive exposure to the sun. If you have very fair, sunsensitive skin and are crazy to join the "summer crowd," I'd say give it a shot. In most men, the result of this internal tanning will be possibly a bit better than what they would get from a bronzer. The primary ingredient in the best of these capsules is something called canthaxanthin, a carotenoid nutrient similar to beta-carotene, the vegetable form of vitamin A. Taken internally, the canthaxanthin gradually darkens your skin. It is better than a bronzer because it does afford you some protection from sun damage, and the carotene element has been hailed by doctors as a possible safeguard against some types of cancer. All in all, I'd say this product is the best for any man who wants a tan but must avoid the sun. Most of these capsules are pretty expensive, but if some kind of tan is a must, they might be worth the price.

Weather Effects

Question: I think I've cornered the market on chapped lips. Is there any masculine way to get rid of the problem?

The easiest and most effective way to combat chapped lips is to carry a Chapstick in your pocket and use it as often as necessary. I know a lot of men feel uneasy using a Chapstick because it reminds them of a woman's lipstick. Come on! Real men do eat quiche, and they do use Chapstick. It is, after all, for comfort rather than decorative purposes, and you're not required to apply it with the aid of a compact mirror. Chapped lips are caused by a combination of sun, wind, and cold, and they can become annoying to you and the women in your life. How would you like to give a big moist kiss to the outside of a pineapple?

Question: My skin seems to get oily in the summer and dry in the winter. Can weather have a big effect on skin?

Even climate has a tremendous effect on the skin. In one degree or another, nearly every man's skin reacts to seasonal changes the way yours does. It's a fact that people who live in parts of the world that have moist, temperate climates with less sunlight have generally better complexions than those who have to face the batterings of extreme changes in the weather. The sun is the most potent dryer and dehydrator of the human skin, but wind and cold weather can also do that job. Interestingly, a particularly dry winter skin may be caused by something happening inside your house or apartment rather than outdoors. Central heating during the winter can cause your skin to become unusually dry. A humidifier can help ease the problem.

Working Out

> *Question*: My work doesn't give me the time for daily running or involvement in regular sports, but I do work out at a health club three times a week. Can the weight machines have any effect on my skin, pro or con?

If you grunt and grimace too much as you increase the amount of weight you can manipulate, you run the risk of carving wrinkles into your face. You should always apply a good covering of water and an invisible moisturizer immediately before you do any such strenuous exercise. Weight machines have been a real boon for those who want to keep their bodies in trim while expending a minimum amount of time. They are great for maintaining both skin and muscle tone on the overall body. They do very little for the face and could induce some problems if attacked too vigorously. Remember, laughing and frowning are the two greatest implanters of facial wrinkles on men with drying or aging skin.

> *Question*: My health club has a sauna and a steam bath. Everyone says they're great although I don't like them that much. Are they good or bad for the skin?

Medically, the jury is still out. In my opinion, extremes of heat and cold are both potentially damaging to the skin if you have a sensitive face. The curative claims for all that incredible heat, particularly in a sauna, are mind-boggling and generally unprovable. Younger men with normal or combination skin will suffer little skin damage if they find either or both baths relaxing or otherwise physically helpful. The 180 to 190 degree heat and almost absent humidity of a sauna might provide some benefit for men with dry skin by encouraging the sebaceous glands to work harder. Always apply a moisturizer afterward. By the same token, a sauna might aggravate the problems of men with oily skin. They should be careful to clean and exfoliate carefully afterward to avoid clogged pores. If you like to use both sauna and steam bath, I would suggest saving the steam for last. The great danger is from dehydration, and that can really wreck your face. Try it if you must, but pay attention to what it may be doing to your face, and do not overdo it.

Sportsman's Face—Quick Menu

1. Strenuous exercise is excellent for the skin, but it can also lead to dehydration. Be prepared to moisturize.
2. Overexposure to the sun can be devastating to your skin.
3. Never sunbathe between the hours of 10:00 A.M. and 2:00 P.M.
4. Everyone should use a sunscreen lotion, graded according to the amount of protection you need.
5. Fair-skinned men with dry, dehydrated, or aging skin should avoid the sun or use a protective sun-blocking lotion.
6. Rushing a tan invariably leads to burning and is highly damaging to every skin type.
7. Any outdoor sport or work can lead to skin damage from the sun, wind, weather, and pollutants. Protectants and moisturizers must be remembered.
8. Sand, water, and snow are natural reflectors that increase the potency of the sun's ultraviolet rays.
9. Follow directions when using tanning lights.
10. Visored caps and proper sunglasses can protect the skin, hair, and eyes during golf and other outdoor sports.
11. Chapped lips can be overcome with the unembarrassed use of Chapstick.
12. Moisturize before and after heavy weight workouts in gyms and health clubs.
13. Saunas and steam baths can be harmful for men with dry and oily skin. Approach with caution.

6

Depression of the Thirties and Beyond: Aging Skin

Let's face it—there is only one fool-proof way to avoid aging: die young! Anyone who tells you otherwise is speaking with forked tongue. That's the bad news. The good news is that you can escape many of the problems of aging skin by beginning a sensible skin care program while you're young and continuing to follow it for the rest of your life. Even better news, if you're already into your forties and beyond, is that you can keep what you've got and minimize further deterioration.

Biologically, there's no way of getting completely around the fact that every man's oil glands get a little lazier with each year he adds to his life. Fortunately, we can do a pretty good job of making up for this loss of natural moisture by doing it ourselves. Any man who begins to notice a drying of his skin and telltale lines must start using moisturizers.

> *Question*: I'm in my fifties, I've got plenty of wrinkles, and I've been married to the same woman for over twenty-five years. Are you going to tell me I've got to climb into bed with her with slippery glop all over my face every night?

Answer: No! And with a little luck your wife will also
be free of facial goo and hair curlers. That sort
of stuff should be reserved for old marital cartoons.

I think it's those old cartoons depicting a fat wife slathered in
grease and with her hair resembling a communications satellite that
many men think about when they hear the word *moisturizer*. The
word still has an unfortunate feminine ring to it because women
were the only ones to take advantage of moisturizers until recent
years. Modern research and technology has given us new products,
specifically designed for men, that should be acceptable to anyone,
no matter how macho he may be.

The Truth About Moisturizers for Men

A loss of natural skin moisture has nothing to do with gender.
Replenishing that supply of moisture makes good sense for everyone. Because of the stigma attached to all face creams as something
that only women use, most men feel more comfortable using a
product that was clearly designed for men. The manufacturers are
aware of this, and the masculine packaging is going to cost you
more. In many cases the results you get are no better than what
you could have gotten from your girlfriend's moisturizer or one of
the inexpensive commercial products that don't attempt to identify
the potential buyer. The one obvious preference in sticking with a
man's product, especially for daytime use, is that a man doesn't
want the stuff to show or smell once he's got it on.

It's important to remember that the moisturizer you purchase
doesn't need to do the actual job of moisturizing the skin. Its
primary function is merely to hold in the water you apply to the
dry areas of your face. If you sleep alone and don't care about
aesthetics, you could simply spray your face with water before
retiring and cover it with a thin coat of plain old Vaseline rubbed
deeply into the skin.

The point is, you need a moisturizer only because you are getting a bit older or are afflicted by dry or dehydrated skin caused by
other factors. You've probably been slapping a drying after-shave
lotion on your face all your adult life. Simply alter the routine and

use a really beneficial moisturizer in its place. You want to use a product that will remain invisible to touch and sight once it's applied and one that will help restore what nature has taken away. A full line of men's moisturizers can be found at all good drug and department stores. If you have dry, dehydrated, or aging skin, a good men's moisturizer may prove to be the most valuable thing in your bathroom cabinet.

Solving the Mystery of Misting

If you have skin that is highly susceptible to aging, no matter the date on your birth certificate, you must keep it as well watered as a hothouse plant. It's the water rather than the store-bought moisturizer that your skin craves. The daily washing and bathing takes care of a bit of the problem, but you must mist the face as often as possible and then apply the moisturizer to make up for what the weather has swiped and what your sebaceous glands can't supply.

In this instance, I'm going to give you a little extra homework to keep you from forgetting this great tool in the fight against aging skin. Find yourself an empty glass bottle with a spray top. The kind some window cleaners come in would suit the purpose. Here's the routine:

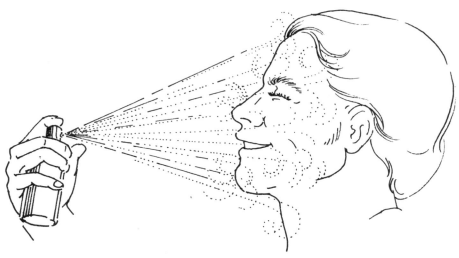

Using spray moisturizer

Spray Misting Preparation

1. Sterilize spray bottle and cap in boiling water for approximately ten minutes.
2. Fill spray bottle with Mountain Valley Water, seal, and spray on face. Do not dry.
3. Cover with fine coat of men's moisturizer.
4. Repeat at least three times daily.

If you're really lazy and don't want to fiddle with preparing the spray bottle, you can simply use the finest spray possible on your shower head. Once you get into the routine, this procedure will really help dry or dehydrated skin, no matter what your actual age is. If you're already past the age of forty, it will soon make your face softer and more pliable, and you'll be much less susceptible to wrinkling.

> *Rule*:   Misting and moisturizing are the only natural ways of forestalling the ravages of aging skin.

Aging Skin Problems

> *Question*: Okay, I'll do it! I'm in my forties, but I think the condition of my neck gives away my age more than my face. What causes it and what can I do about it?

Work at it because you are not alone. The neck is a special problem area for men with aging skin, more so than with women. Men usually forget about their necks whereas women don't. Did you ever wonder about those sharp-looking caps the soldiers wore in all the films about the French Foreign Legion? They had the standard French Army kepi with a flowing white scarf attached to the back. That white thing was to protect the back of the neck from the hot rays of the desert sun. Many of us forget about the backs of our necks when we apply sunscreen or moisturizer. Too many of us also fail to recognize that the front of the neck is usually a dry area that needs moisturizing. Always spray and moisturize the neck, front and back, when you do your face. Later in this chapter I'll give specific exercises that will also help you maintain muscle and skin tone in this area.

> *Question*: I'm in my late forties, and I'll admit I haven't taken great care of my skin, especially in regard to the sun. I started noticing a few brown spots on my hands about a year ago, and now I see a couple high on my forehead. Can these be age spots?

Some people call them that, but your condition proves they don't have much to do with old age. Others call them liver spots, and they don't have anything to do with the liver, except for a similarity in color. The medical term is *lentigo*, and these brown spots are another result of long-term overexposure to the sun. If you have the time and the patience, it's possible to bleach them somewhat with a number of home preparations including lemon juice. Here's a situation where I'd recommend paying a visit to a dermatologist. Dermatologists can make them effectively disappear with a treatment that utilizes dry ice. The treatment is painless, fast, and relatively inexpensive. An older man competing with younger guys for jobs or feminine favors might find the doctor's visit very worthwhile.

> *Question*: A few months ago I noticed that I could suddenly see what looks like a lot of little veins on and near my nose. I'm fifty-eight. Does the skin get thinner when you age?

In a sense it does because its support system is breaking down. However, the condition you are describing is something called couperose skin. Those are veins you're noticing, and the problem will probably get worse without proper treatment. It's a common problem among older men, particularly those who have spent a lot of time outdoors in extreme weather. Couperose skin does nothing for your good looks and can be an indication of more serious trouble such as circulatory problems and possible heart disease. For that reason you should see a doctor as soon as possible. A good dermatologist can correct the situation, if it's only a skin problem, by using a needle or a dry ice treatment similar to that used to correct lentigo.

Question: A friend of mine—we're both in our mid forties—got about forty pounds overweight. He wanted to get in shape for the summer and managed to take the excess off in about three months. Now his face looks really ancient and saggy. Is dieting bad for the skin?

A quick weight-loss diet can be disastrous for the skin. You are describing another common problem found among middle-aged men who are basically sedentary and become suddenly panic-stricken about looking old. The face is almost always the first thing to suffer. Many fast diets really reduce body weight by dehydration more than anything else. You dehydrate your skin along with the rest of your body, and you can cause permanent damage to your face by depleting the collagen of the dermis which gives your outer skin its support. Coupled with the normal dryness of aging skin and the working of gravity, that kind of weight loss can lead to sagging facial skin, creases, and deep folds. Nothing, except maybe a sharp scalpel, can create overnight wonders in the areas of weight loss or skin rejuvenation. Good information, patience, and perseverance are the keys to real success.

Question: I'm only thirty-five, but it looks to me like I'm starting to get bags under my eyes. My dad has them, and I wonder if they're hereditary. Can you do anything about them?

There's no doubt that bags under the eyes are almost as vexing a problem as thinning hair. Like balding, some of the problem can be blamed on heredity, and there isn't a great deal you can do about the problem on your own. That's why it's important for younger men to take special care of the eye area before bags have a chance to form. The skin around the eyes is very thin, with virtually no support under the epidermis. Men of all ages should make certain they keep the area above and below the eyes well moisturized. Facial exercises (coming up) can also be of help, and many doctors advise sleeping with the head slightly elevated to cause the fluid to drain better. Cold compresses can ease temporary swelling, but there's little you can do at home to really rid yourself of the problem. Droopy, baggy eyes can really age a man's face, but you may not want to run out to see a plastic surgeon until you have exhausted every other option.

Facial Exercises Can Work for You

Facial exercise is often the court of last resort for men with saggy, aging skin, and that's why I have included it in this chapter. However, facial exercise is not just for older men. Ideally, everyone should practice these easy movements, not waiting until the natural moisturizing wanes and aging begins. Exercise and body fitness among the knowledgeable has almost reached the point of becoming a national craze. Unfortunately, too few people—professionals and laymen—have examined the long-term benefits to be had from direct exercise of the face.

It isn't because the facial areas have no muscles. The face and neck are laced with muscle fibers; otherwise, we would be unable to laugh, cry, chew, or even spit. Take a moment to study the medical illustration of the muscles of the face and neck. It's these neglected muscles that we want to exercise, muscles that can have a profound effect on the way your face will look as you reach your middle years and beyond.

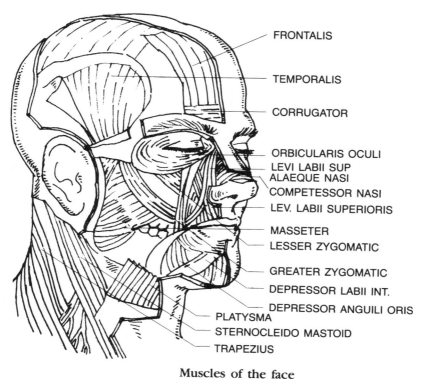

FRONTALIS

TEMPORALIS

CORRUGATOR

ORBICULARIS OCULI
LEVI LABII SUP
ALAEQUE NASI
COMPETESSOR NASI
LEV. LABII SUPERIORIS

MASSETER
LESSER ZYGOMATIC

GREATER ZYGOMATIC
DEPRESSOR LABII INT.
DEPRESSOR ANGUILI ORIS
PLATYSMA
STERNOCLEIDO MASTOID
TRAPEZIUS

Muscles of the face

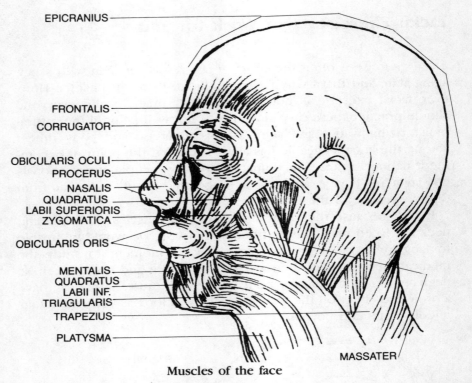

EPICRANIUS

FRONTALIS
CORRUGATOR

OBICULARIS OCULI
PROCERUS
NASALIS
QUADRATUS
LABII SUPERIORIS
ZYGOMATICA

OBICULARIS ORIS

MENTALIS
QUADRATUS
LABII INF.
TRIAGULARIS
TRAPEZIUS

PLATYSMA

MASSATER

Muscles of the face

These muscles, particularly those around the eyes, chin, and neck, are vitally important in preserving the good skin tone of the face and neck. They're obviously small muscles compared to those you have elsewhere, but they can be tightened and developed in the exact same way, and that will lead to a remarkable improvement in your skin. The skin and flesh of your bicep looks far less saggy and flabby after you've worked out with weights. Your facial skin and flesh will respond with equal enthusiasm to facial exercise.

Facial exercise is both preventive and corrective. Like every other aspect of my skin care program, the sooner you start these exercises, the better your chances of keeping your skin and muscle tone youthful throughout your life. Patient adherence to this workout will help you make up for lost time. Facial muscles will respond, no matter what your age, and you will be rewarded with better condition and tone after several weeks. Obviously, older men will take longer to show improvement, just as it takes some of us longer to get into overall physical shape. The results will not be instantaneous, and exercise will do little to firm the face if you are grossly overweight with fatty deposits that cause bulging cheeks and double chins. On the other hand, unlike pushups and other exercises to build the body, these activities for the face are neither difficult nor tiring and can be done almost anywhere at your own convenience.

If you've wondered why so many of your favorite male stars of movies and television seem never to age, it's because many of them religiously follow this same program of facial exercise. Perry King, macho blond star of a top-rated NBC adventure series, regularly exercises his face this way, with special emphasis on the neck area, where most men first begin to show the signs of aging. Of course, Perry is a young man gifted with good skin, but it is never too early—or too late—to benefit from this program.

These exercises tone and tighten rather than stretch and weaken. I want to emphasize that I agree with other skin experts who say it is not good to stretch or put undo pressure on the facial skin because that kind of action could lead to a weakening of the connective tissue below the epidermis. The facial exercises I'm suggesting will have the opposite effect. My program will give you the advantage of skin massage while you tone and tighten the facial muscles. A good example of the benefits of exercise and massage is something we do every day without thinking about it. Have you noticed that very few men, whatever their age, have deep wrinkling around the lips the way some women do? One of the chief reasons for this is that men shave and women don't. We go through some unplanned, and sometimes grotesque exercises in order to get our pelts in position to be shaved. The shaving actually acts as a massage, and we end up with fewer deep lines around the lips.

Again, the biggest problems for men—usually the first to betray our age—are puffiness around the eyes, sagging jowls, and what could be called turkey neck. Misting and moisturizing, along with great respect for the destructive power of the sun, will help prevent these problems. Regular massage and facial exercise will also stall the forces of gravity and restore much of the skin and muscle tone of your youth. In the interest of your valuable time, I have designed most of these exercises to be performed under your own shower while you have a fine mist on your face. If your face is properly moisturized, these exercises can be done almost any place and at any time.

The Shower As Gymnasium: Facial Exercises

For Double Chin

Lean the head back as far as possible into the spray; bring the bottom lip up over the top lip, attempting to touch your nose. Do this very slowly and hold, then release and come back down slowly into the starting position. Do this at least five times daily, always with very slow and deliberate movement that will tighten the muscles rather than stretch the skin.

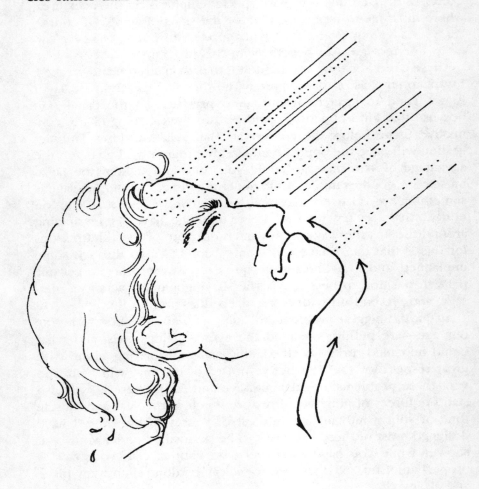

For the Neck

This exercise can be done on couch or bed. Lie flat on back with head extended off bed or couch. Raise head slowly to horizontal position while slowly extending bottom lip over top lip, as in previous exercise, trying to touch your nose. Hold, then slowly lower head and bottom lip to starting position. Do at least five times daily.

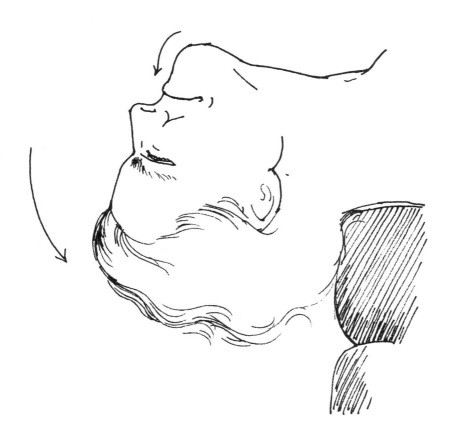

For Chin and Jawline

Can be done any place. With mouth closed, move the tip of your tongue down and backward in an almost swallowing movement. Repeat slowly five times to strengthen muscles in lower face and neck.

For the Jowls

With the head in vertical position, again bring bottom lip over top lip and try to smile broadly in the direction of the right eye. Come back to starting position and repeat procedure on left side. Make movement slow and deliberate, and repeat five times.

For Eye Bags

Take your index fingers and place them at the very corner of each eye. Gently pull the skin and muscle to the side, no more than an eighth of an inch, and slowly close your eyes. Slowly release tension and reopen eyes. Repeat at least five times.

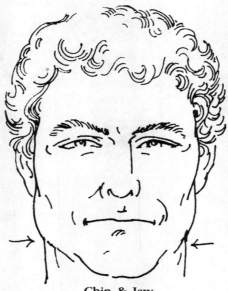

Chin & Jaw

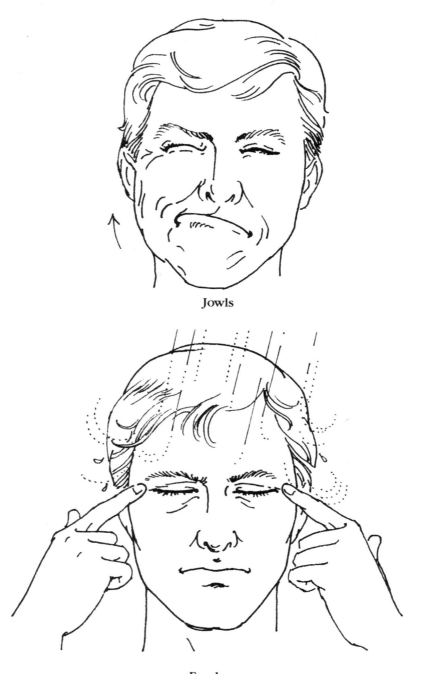

Jowls

Eye bags

For Droopy Eyelids

Cup hands to keep water from stinging eyes, and place three middle fingers directly under each eyebrow. Push gently upward as far as comfortable, then slowly close eyes. The slower the movement, the more tension you place on the muscles. Repeat at least five times.

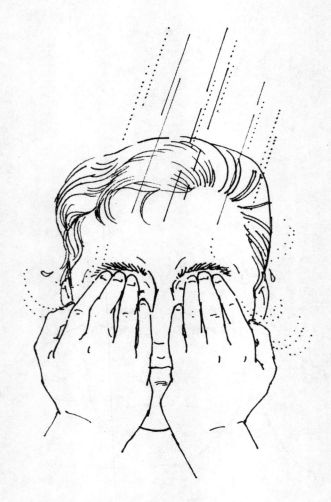

Droopy eyelids

As you can see, we're not talking Arnold Schwarzenegger here. These exercises are ridiculously simple, require little discipline, and will plant no bulging muscles on your kisser. When practiced during your shower while you rinse off the soap, they will keep your facial muscles and skin in fine tone and either obviate or delay the need for more drastic measures. It's important to remember that exercise will not remove herniated fat around the eyes, nor will it cause you to look twenty years younger overnight. Facial exercise is no panacea. But it should be an integral part of your complete skin care program which will keep you ahead in the battle against drooping, sagging, aging skin.

Is Plastic Surgery a Masculine Option?

A recent nationwide survey indicated that more than two-thirds of American men over the age of thirty-five believe it is. In face-to-face interviews conducted by a respected marketing research organization, these men fully approved of surgical procedures that could correct signs of aging and give a man more self-esteem and a better opportunity for career advancement. Statistics confirm the viewpoint of the survey, with plastic surgery operations up 61 percent between 1981 and 1984. In some of the major metropolitan areas, as many as 40 percent of these operations are performed on men. That's a huge shift from even a decade ago, when perhaps only 10 percent of cosmetic surgery patients were male.

At the very beginning I emphasized that I had no intention of giving you a "beauty book" for men. My aim has not changed in the slightest, because my experience has convinced me that most men can maintain a good-looking and basically youthful skin throughout their lifetimes, providing they work at good skin care. However, nothing I or anyone else can teach you will correct problems that are hereditary or the result of decades of abuse and neglect. If you have failed to correct the problem in time, only surgery will help. I am not going to talk about nose jobs, chin augmentation, liposuction, or other cosmetic procedures that have to do with obvious vanity. I do think it is important to give you information on surgical procedures that will erase the years that home practice can't change.

Nearly every reputable plastic surgeon will tell you that the increase in male patients has more to do with job competition than with vanity. We are living in the most youth-oriented society in the history of humanity, and that thinking has had its most traumatic effect on the job market where past forty too often means over the hill to those who hand out the promotions or do the hiring. That kind of corporate thinking was one of the reasons for this book. There is no valid reason for any dynamic man to allow an aging face to camouflage a vigorous mind.

I do feel that plastic surgery is a viable option for any man—as a last resort. In later chapters I'll discuss surgical procedures for unusual skin problems and for loss of hair. By and large, I think an older man should have no reluctance to consider the possibility of cosmetic surgery to correct two areas that home care might have prevented if caught in time. These operations, in order of importance, are:

1. Blepharoplasty
2. Rhytidectomy

Interestingly, these two operations are already the ones most often requested by men. The first is a procedure that corrects droopy, baggy eyes, and the second is what is commonly known as a face lift. I have no hesitation about recommending these operations for older men who feel they would benefit from them. If older men have really deep bags under their eyes or heavy skin folds, home care can do relatively little to correct the problem.

The Facts About Plastic Surgery

A well-known surgeon at California's Stanford University says men rarely show up at his office with a picture of a movie star and say, "Make me look like him." Most men only want to look like themselves, the way they did a few years earlier. That is why, when you're certain it's too late to do it yourself, you should feel no less masculine when you turn to a plastic surgeon. If looking younger is really important to your mental well-being or career goals, go for it.

The two surgical procedures I would recommend for older men whose faces have gone beyond the reach of home maintenance are not going to drastically alter your appearance. They will simply correct the worst effects of droopy eyelids and bags under the eyes in the eye operation, and smooth away the most noticeable sags in the face lift. Few older men would be happy about the prospects of facing a barrage of questions if they were to return to the office looking twenty years younger. Most men do look better with a few hard-earned character lines in their faces. I would suggest the face lift only for an older man who, for business or very personal reasons, wants to remove really bad sagging that makes him look older than his years. The jowls and neck are particularly troublesome areas that can be improved. Correcting the eye area alone will give a man a vital new look which will erase the misleading message that he is burned-out, old, and tired.

If you feel the need to undergo plastic surgery, you must go about selecting a surgeon in a very businesslike manner. Your skin care program, to this point, has cost you only the price of this book. Plastic surgery can cost big bucks, and there are wild fluctuations among the fees of the doctors. Money, of course, should not be the primary consideration; finding a skilled surgeon with whom you can relate is far more important. Plastic surgery is an art as well as a science. You want a Michelangelo rather than a Picasso. Communication is vitally important, so don't be timid about shopping around.

Blepharoplasty

This is a surgically simple operation but one that can, by itself, give a man a subtly youthful appearance. Aging causes the upper eyelids to droop, effectively taking away the wide-eyed look of youth and causing the formation of bags under the eyes. This operation solves both problems and takes a relatively short amount of time. The surgeon trims away the loose skin and also removes the patches of fat that have collected to cause the baggy look. If you prefer, you can find a doctor who will perform the surgery right in his or her office, and you can recuperate in the privacy of your own home. Dark glasses will allow you to walk around outdoors without undo staring, but you should plan on being absent from work for at least two weeks until the swelling and bruising disappear. The cost of a blepharoplasty can range anywhere from $600 to $4,000.

Rhytidectomy

This so-called face lift operation is second in popularity among men because it can correct a number of major skin problems brought on by neglect and abuse. It is particularly effective for older men because it can greatly improve the appearance of the jowls and neck. A face lift is also a far more complicated and lengthy operation than an "eye job." A face lift can, at the surgeon's discretion, be performed in an office surgical suite or in a hospital. The operation usually lasts from two to three hours, but the patient feels no discomfort under either a local or general anesthetic. Most doctors prefer a hospitalization of only three to four days. The procedure consists of making incisions in the temple and around the ear and upper neck and actually lifting the skin, redraping, and tightening it before stitching it back into place. This operation will not erase all the deep wrinkles of your face, but it will take away most of the heavy folds and sagging of the cheeks, jowls, and neck. Your hospitalization will be brief, but it's unlikely you would want anyone but your family or closest friends to get a peek at you for at least two weeks until the most obvious bruising and swelling have disappeared. Unless you've advised everyone of your plans, it may be as long as three weeks before you'll feel comfortable returning to work with your rejuvenated face. Rhytidectomies are considerably more costly than blepharoplasties and range in price from $1,500 to $8,000. If you feel the need for both operations, it would be better to have them done at the same time. That would save you both money and time away from work.

Obviously, the decision to undergo plastic surgery is not one that should be taken lightly. The two I have described are safe, painless operations, but they are expensive and require an extended period of isolation if you intend to keep your "home improvement" strictly private. A simple test to see if you are a good candidate for such surgery can be performed at home. Look at yourself in the mirror and place three fingers of each hand at the sideburn area on each side of your face. Now push gently and see how much difference the new tension makes. Don't push hard enough to distort your features. If what you see is a decided improvement, and nothing else seems to be working, you should start checking for a dependable, compatible plastic surgeon.

Aging Skin—Quick Menu

1. Any man with dry, dehydrated, or aging skin, regardless of age, must start using moisturizers.

2. Men should use moisturizers that are nongreasy, nonsticky, and completely invisible after they are applied.

3. Water actually moisturizes the skin, the moisturizer only keeps the water locked in.

4. A spray mist is best for coating the face, through the suggested spray bottle or a special shower head.

5. The neck is a particular problem area for older men. Keep it well moisturized and exercised.

6. Lentigo, brown spots on face and hands, are caused by years of overexposure to the sun. Home remedies and over-the-counter bleaching products work slowly. A dermatologist can get rid of them quickly with a dry ice treatment.

7. Couperose skin, the appearance of tiny veins in the face, can be an indication of serious medical problems and calls for a visit to a doctor. He or she can alleviate the problem with office treatment.

8. Quick weight loss diets are a no-no for men with aging skin. This kind of diet causes dehydration that ravages both the dermis and epidermis, which alters the facial structure and brings on heavy sagging.

9. The skin above and below the eyes is the thinnest and least protected on a man's face. Only long-term care and lucky genes can prevent deterioration into droopy, baggy eyes. Keep well moisturized and protected from the sun.

10. Facial exercises, outlined in this chapter, are an excellent at-home preventive for saggy skin on the neck and other fragile parts of the face.

11. If you've passed the point of no return regarding eyes, jowls, and neck, plastic surgery is your best alternative. The appropriate operations are called blepharoplasty (eye job) and rhytidectomy (face lift).

12. Communication, performance, and fees fluctuate wildly among plastic surgeons. Shop around until you find the one that best suits your individual needs.

7

The Pits: Acne and Other Special Problems

As I said at the beginning, this book has been specifically designed to provide you with the information you will need to keep your skin smooth and healthy in the convenience and privacy of your own home. However, because of heredity and other factors, many men develop special problems that sometimes get out of control. A list of Latin names of some typical skin disorders—Milia, Comedones, Seborrhea, Streatoma, Furuncle—sounds like something to be found in a catalogue of expensive Italian sports cars. Of course, these disturbances are anything but amusing to the man who suffers from them.

I've spent a great portion of this book stressing the importance of preserving the natural oils and moisture of the face as an effective means of combatting the natural aging process. But some men have a surplus of sebum early in their adulthood, and most of the skin disorders listed above—and others—are caused by workaholic oil glands. While naturally oily skin can keep us looking younger than our contemporaries, it can also cause problems that will plague us for the rest of our lives. These problems are not easily cured, certainly not in the pages of a book, and direct visits to a dermatologist or professional esthetician are advised. However, knowledge is power. Understanding the problem, its cause and possible cure, is a good starting point in your struggle to rid yourself of it.

Debunking the Myths About Acne

There is probably nothing more psychologically painful for a young man attempting to gain confidence in dealing with the opposite sex than to come down with a severe case of acne. Most of us outgrow the worst stages of it by our early twenties, but the psychological and sometimes physical scars linger on. As in the case of the common cold, medical science has not yet developed a sure-fire cure.

We have progressed in the treatment for this embarrassing skin problem in recent years, and it is now far easier to keep it under some kind of control. That's a far better situation than not too long ago, when a face full of unsightly blemishes caused many to believe that the victim either did not spend proper time on personal hygiene or continually pigged out on chocolate or greasy foods. As it happens, none of these old wives' tales about the causes and treatment of acne have more than a grain of truth in them.

Sadly, there are still more sound theories about acne than established facts. We do know that acne is a problem that affects most people at the onset of puberty, it is usually related to hormonal changes in the body, it goes hand in hand (or cheek and jowl) with overactive sebaceous glands, and it is often hereditary. That leaves us with very little control. We can't do anything about our heredity, and we must wait for the hormonal changes to run their course. The one area where we can exert some strong influence is in the matter of the excessively oily skin.

Here's how the condition develops. You're a normal, happy teenager who is beginning to get over the embarrassment of your voice changing. You're planning to make some highly sophisticated moves in the direction of a special classmate. You've already started shaving despite your dad's insistence that it isn't necessary. It doesn't matter because you know you are a man, in fact if not in age. Then you wake up one morning to discover a huge red pimple on your chin. Before long you have more and more of the same kind of pimples, and the condition continues throughout high school and on into college. At the very time you need to look your best, you feel like some kind of freak.

Did you bring it on yourself? In most cases, you probably did not. If either of your parents suffered from it in their adolescence, they may have inadvertently passed it on to you. But all is not lost. Acne is not an almost hopeless situation, such as inherited baldness. In strictly biological terms, your problem probably started with a common blackhead, and we can successfully keep those in check. Ironically, nearly all acne outbreaks start with blackheads, although not everyone with blackheads will develop acne. If you begin careful skin care at the outset of acne, there's an excellent possibility that you will be able to keep it under control.

Since nearly every pimple grows from a blackhead, it is our first order of business to keep the face clear of those smaller blemishes. Remember our earlier section on the care of very oily skin? It's the surplus sebum that creates blackheads by clogging the pores, solidifying, and turning dark. It's imperative that you adhere to a daily regimen of care for men with oily skin. This is infinitely more important if you have noticed that pimples and blackheads are more than just occasional annoyances. In other words, you will have to work harder at your skin care program than other men until you outgrow the condition that makes you prone to acne.

1. Thoroughly cleanse the face with an appropriate soap in the morning, after work, and before retiring.
2. Exfoliate the skin with each washing to rid it of the dead particles that can lead to clogged pores.

Because of the mystifying nature of acne, this extra care will not ensure that you will be completely free of the problem. But it will help you to keep it under control. The old idea of using calamine lotion and strong astringents is not entirely in favor today. In fact, we know it's dangerous to overdo drying the skin because the sebaceous glands of acne-prone men often work overtime, frantically producing more oil in direct proportion with your attempt to slow them down. Regular washings with a good soap are your best bet. Most commercial astringents with fancy names and price tags to match are primarily composed of alchohol or witch hazel. Both are obviously quite capable of ridding the skin of surplus oil, but you would be as well off buying the generic stuff. Again, if you have some regular after-shave lotion on the bathroom shelf, it will serve the purpose of an astringent if you feel the need of one. Pay careful attention to see if it is actually doing the job intended.

By all means, continue to clean and exfoliate your skin. Getting those dead cells cleared away before they inflict the maximum damage is the surest way to keep acne under control. Work very gingerly around the major blemishes, and be certain to use a clean brush or washcloth every time to avoid spreading germs and infection.

> *Rule*: Avoid squeezing or picking at pimples and black-heads. Improper procedure will spread the infection and possibly result in permanent scarring.

If your acne condition is really bad, with large pustules obviously ripe for the breaking, you would be far better off consulting a dermatologist or professional esthetician. The risks in doing it yourself are simply too great. Fortunately, newly developed drugs are proving to be wonderfully successful in treating acne conditions. By all means, don't give up! Work at your home program if your case is mild or past its peak, or see a doctor. The longer acne goes unattended, the longer it will stay with you.

I have deliberately avoided giving you much in the way of home remedies, facials, and that sort of thing because I recognize that most men simply do not have the time or patience for such things. However, acne is such a disturbing problem that any young man who has it is probably going to be willing to take as much time as necessary to rid himself of it. In this special case, I will suggest a home remedy and facial procedure that does get results, depending on the severity of the condition. It requires minimum time and effort.

Home Acne Treatment

1. The face must be thoroughly cleaned and exfoliated in the manner suggested for oily skin, morning and evening.
2. A special home facial must be applied at least twice each week.
3. Mix one tablespoon of baking soda in one pint of Mountain Valley Water to form a lotion.

4. Saturate clean cotton pads with this disincrustation lotion and place on areas of newly cleaned skin that show acne eruptions.
5. Leave the saturated compresses on the enlarged follicles, blemishes, and blackheads for a full 15 minutes.
6. Remove the lotion using fresh cotton pads soaked in cool water, and gently massage area with fingertips for approximately five minutes.

This home facial is not a cure-all for serious acne, but it is comparable to the treatment given in the best professional skin care salons and should be a definite help in controlling your problem. Most of us outgrow the worst effects of acne in our early twenties, but any young man who has a serious case would benefit from a visit to his family doctor or a dermatologist.

> *Question*: Does diet have no effect at all on acne? I'm still bothered by it, and I've heard that seafood makes it worse. Is that true?

The entire business of diet and acne is still very much up in the air, but the medical profession has determined that too much iodine in the diet can cause a bad reaction in men who are acne prone. Most doctors have no bias against seafood in general, but they will advise you to avoid all shellfish—shrimp, lobster, etc. If you are trying to rid yourself of acne, it might be advisable to switch temporarily to a noniodized table salt. Some acne sufferers are not at all affected by iodine intake, and, since a certain amount is essential to your overall health, careful experimentation is desirable.

> *Question*: Is Vitamin E a kind of wonder drug for acne as some people claim?

Not in my book. Most doctors agree that it does nothing to cure acne, internally or externally. Since it usually comes as an oil in capsule form, it makes little sense to apply more oil to an excessively oily skin. There have been similar claims for the use of vitamin A, but overdosage of vitamin A can be highly dangerous. I believe you would be better served to consult with a physician before experimenting on your own.

Question: Can worry and agitation affect the skin? It seems to me that my face always used to break out in college every time an important exam was scheduled. It still happens, to a lesser degree, when I'm under pressure.

You're right on the money with your assumption. It has been proven that stress is a definite contributor to skin blemishing. I'll go into greater detail about this subject later, but it's interesting that at least one old wives' tale, usually an old coach's tale with men, has a gram of truth in it.

Question: I had very serious acne when I was a kid, and I'm still bothered by occasional pimples. But it's the acne scars on my face that really bug me. Is there any way to get rid of these?

Deep scarring from adolescent acne is the worst problem because these reminders of an insecure adolescence never leave of their own accord. For what it's worth, women who are knowledgeable about the hormonal surge that created the scars consider them proof positive of a man's virility. Of course, this is little comfort to the man who must look at them in the mirror every morning. If you can't live with them, you'd best see a plastic surgeon. Many consider the correcting of acne-scarred skin among cosmetic surgery's most worthwhile achievements.

There are basically three kinds of acne scars: the icepick pore scar, the acne pit scar, and the raised scar. The icepick scar is aptly named because the skin is damaged as if it has been gouged by an ice pick or other narrow instrument, leaving the pore open and deep. The pit scar is perhaps the most common, resulting from a large eruption that has left the tissue shrunken and depressed. The raised scar develops when several large cysts have erupted together in close formation and created a lumpy mass of tissue on the skin. All of these conditions can be greatly improved—sometimes eradicated—by relatively simple procedures in plastic surgery. The procedures are neither painless nor inexpensive, but they can be worthwhile if you are deeply troubled by the reminders of your adolescent acne.

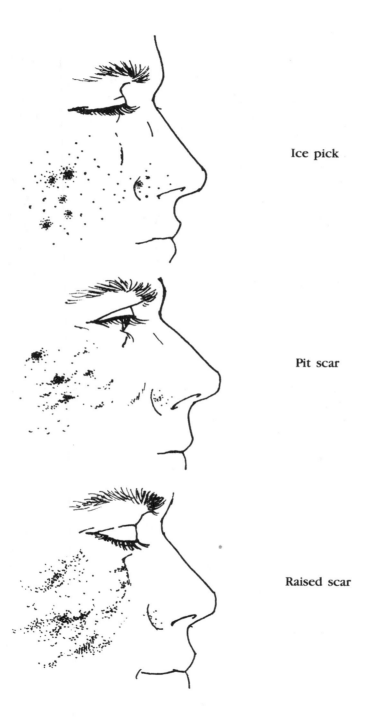

Ice pick

Pit scar

Raised scar

Dermabrasion

This is an office procedure that is best for skin that has wide areas of deep pit scars. The surgeon will take a stainless steel brush, electrically operated, and literally sand away several layers of skin, leaving the final surface as close as possible to the depth of the pit scars. Under a local anesthetic, the procedure is painless, but the recovery can be very unpleasant. Your face will be bandaged immediately after the operation, and you can go home. On the following day the bandages come off and the sanded skin will heal on its own, much the way a badly scraped knee did when you were little. You'll have a face that will frighten your dog for at least two weeks until the crust drops off and the new skin takes its place. Even then you'll have more waiting until you look completely normal. Obviously, the success of the procedure will depend on the depth of your acne scars. Costs for dermabrasion run between $250 and $2,500.

Chemabrasion

This procedure can also be carried out in the doctor's office and operates on the same principle as dermabrasion, except that the surgeon peels off the layers of skin with strong chemicals. Recovery time from this procedure is also two weeks or more, and the costs average about the same as for regular dermabrasion. If you have this type of chemical peeling, your face will be highly photosensitive, and you must stay out of bright sunlight.

Zyderm Injections

This is a relatively new procedure that has had some success in treating acne ice pick scars. Zyderm is a form of collagen that is injected into the scars to plump them up, and the same collagen also has been used with some success to smooth out extra deep wrinkles. Costs for this treatment are comparable to those for the abrasive procedures.

It's important to remember that none of these procedures will be perfect if your acne scarring is very severe. You probably will not have baby-smooth skin after healing. The skin removal operations are not inexpensive, and the recovery can be painful. Remember, if you are self-conscious about acne scars, you are likely to make much more of the situation than anyone you are going to meet. I would suggest you interview a number of surgeons and get the straight poop on your individual needs and the amount of improvement you can expect before you subject yourself to any of these treatments.

> *Question*: I've never had acne but I've always been bothered by blackheads. Does that mean I'm not washing properly?

Not necessarily. The black part of the blackhead is not dirt, as many people believe. Comedones (yes, even these ugly things have a scientific name) are caused by the the Jekyll and Hyde oil gland when the excess oil plugs itself, oxydizes and turns black. You can best avoid them by continuing your program of good cleaning and exfoliating for oily skin. Consider yourself lucky that you haven't developed more serious blemishes.

> *Question*: What's the deal on these facial saunas or steam machines that you can use at home? Aren't they good for the face?

If you happen to have one at your disposal, I'd say go ahead and use it from time to time. Either device will help open the pores of your face and could be useful if you have a special problem with blackheads. On the other hand, the steam from your shower will do the same job, and I am very leery of a do-it-yourself project when it comes to eradicating blackheads or pimples. Spreading infection and possible permanent scarring are too likely to make it safe. If you have difficulty ridding your skin of blackheads despite a good cleaning and exfoliating regimen for oily skin, invest your money in a visit to a skin care professional. I think you'll get better results for the money spent.

> *Question*: Sometimes I get little white bumps on my skin. Is there anything called a whitehead?

In fact, the medical term is the one that sounds like an Italian road race: milia. Here's a case where the trapped sebum, bacteria, and other matter miss a pore opening and simply get trapped under the surface of the skin. They're a special problem because there's no way of dislodging them until the horny growth of epidermis covering them gives away and they become pimples. They're another outgrowth of excessively oily skin and, along with blackheads, pimples, and cysts, form the basis of what can become acne.

> *Question*: Toward the end of last summer I got a little patch on my cheek that suddenly began to fade. That place is still lighter than the rest of my face, even after my tan has disappeared. Any idea what it is?

It sounds like a problem called vitiligo, which means a sudden loss of the cells which give us our skin color. Unfortunately, not even medical science has all the answers about what causes this strange inability to produce melanin. You should see a doctor because the problem sometimes signals trouble with the thyroid and/or the adrenal glands and possibly even pernicious anemia. The condition is treatable by a physician.

> *Question*: I'm in my late twenties, and I seldom drink. But I've still got some kind of weird problem because my nose and the area around it occasionally turn a bright red. I feel like W. C. Fields! What's the cause of this?

Too much steady drinking sometimes brings on a skin problem called rosacea. But that doesn't seem to be the culprit in your case. Rosacea is also caused by overactive oil glands. If you have oily skin, follow the regular routine of cleaning and exfoliation. That should, in time, take care of the problem. Here's another tip: stay clear of highly seasoned foods. They can also aggravate the condition.

> *Question*: I have a mole or something close to one corner of my mouth that makes me very self-conscious. I'm tired of using my standard Abe Lincoln line. Is there some way to get rid of it?

If it bleeds, changes color, or is painful, you should see a doctor immediately. It could be evidence of skin cancer. Chances are, as you describe it, it is probably an ordinary mole. A dermatologist can remove it quickly and painlessly with a local anesthetic in his office. He can either shave it off—which may leave a corresponding surface mark where it was—or burn it away or use a scalpel to cut it out. The last procedure is usually the most satisfactory and will leave hardly any scar when properly sutured. The procedure is relatively inexpensive.

Special Problems—Quick Menu

1. Most men will outgrow the worst stages of acne during their early twenties.

2. Acne is not caused by an overindulgence in chocolate or deep-fried foods.

3. Youthful hormonal changes, heredity, and uncontrolled seba-ceous glands precipitate acne.

4. Acne-prone men must take extra care to follow the cleansing routine for oily skin, especially exfoliation.

5. Overuse of astringents can cause the oil glands to produce still more oil.

6. Severe acne can best be treated by a dermatologist. New drugs are proving to be effective in controlling the problem.

7. Do not pick or squeeze acne eruptions. Leave that job to a professional.

8. Acne scars, depending on their depth, can be removed or greatly relieved by cosmetic surgery procedures called derma-brasion, chemabrasion, and zyderm injections.

9. Blackheads can lead to bigger blemishes and can be avoided by disciplined adherence to the oily-skin cleansing program.

10. Steady drinking and highly seasoned foods can lead to redness of the nose and T zone in a condition called rosacea.

11. Moles that bleed, hurt, or change color could be malignant and should be removed by a doctor.

8

Using Your Head to Save Your Hair

Baldness! The sound of the word is enough to send shivers down the spine of an otherwise macho and well-adjusted young man when he considers it in terms of his own head. The inordinate fear of losing the hair probably predates the Samson story in the Bible. To many men it is an event that is dreaded as much as death and taxes. Fortunately, balding is not necessarily as inevitable. Let me put my cards on the table: there are types of male pattern baldness that are almost impossible to treat, but I am prepared to give you the latest information on available help and a sound program of care and maintenance that will help you keep the amount of hair your heredity decreed you were entitled to have.

Hair care is a natural extension of your skin care program. It's important first to realize that the hair is not really as important in the long run as the smooth base from which it grows. That's why we feel no special sorrow when the barber whacks away and lets it fall freely on the floor. It's literally "hair today, gone tomorrow." The real action is taking place in the skin beneath the hair—the scalp. That is where the hair follicles are, where the growth cells are manufacturing new strands of hair to replace the old. The scalp is skin that requires special care to maintain its good health and ability to produce hair. At the same time, the hair already in place must be handled with care in order to keep its good looks and longevity.

Young men of the 1960s and 1970s took hairstyles to extremes not reached since the eighteenth century, but the exuberance of youth has always made it seem that what was growing on top of the head was far more important than any calculated, long-term planning about how to keep it there. Many males of the baby boom now realize that planning might have allowed them to keep more of the luxurious growths they sported fifteen or twenty years ago. The good news is that it's not too late. The more we know about our hair, what helps and hurts it, the sooner we can start our battle to keep it waving.

Hair: What It Is and How It Works

One of the most comforting things to remember is that the hair we see on any male's head—even the luxuriant, impenetrable forest atop the skull of a healthy teenager—is really dead material. From a purely biological viewpoint, like the top layer of the epidermis or the ends of our fingernails, it's already on its way out. Conversely, aesthetic and psychological considerations demand that we do anything except forget about it and let it take its own course.

The logical first step in good hair care is a working knowledge of the scalp. It is composed of epidermis, dermis, and hypodermis already reviewed here. The one major difference between the scalp and other areas of the human skin is that the dermis of the scalp contains many more hair follicles. It also has pores, sweat and sebaceous glands, nerves, and blood vessels. For this reason, it suffers from similar problems and deserves much the same treatment as other parts of the face. However, the hair of the scalp differs from facial or body hair.

Each strand of hair on your head is 97 percent protein and is made up of three layers called the cuticle, the cortex, and the medulla. The individual hair grows from a follicle in the scalp and receives its nourishment from the circulatory system through a microscopic nipple called the papilla. This papilla, at the bottom of the follicle recess, is the hair's true root and will continue to

Human Hair

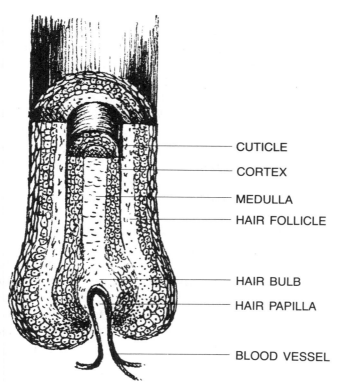

- CUTICLE
- CORTEX
- MEDULLA
- HAIR FOLLICLE

- HAIR BULB
- HAIR PAPILLA

- BLOOD VESSEL

Cross Section

replace old strands while it remains healthy. Each follicle produces only one strand of hair at a time. But, to give you an idea of how many of these follicles are centered in the dermis of the scalp, the average man in his late twenties will have more than 100,000 separate strands of hair growing from his scalp. Interestingly, blond men will have normally several thousand more hairs than brunets, and red-haired men will have a few thousand fewer. From nature's viewpoint, human hair is a covering to protect the top of the head. Redheads require fewer hairs because their individual strands are somewhat more thick. Blond hair strands are generally thinner, accounting for the greater number of them.

How the Hair Grows

Hair growth is known to take place in cycles that are slowed as a man ages. A single strand of hair is normally so thin that science has done its research in measurements almost beyond our comprehension. Hair actually gets thinner with age, thinner in the sense of individual strand diameter rather than head cover. Hair diameter is measured in microns, units that equal millionths of a meter. An individual strand of hair will lose two to three microns of thickness with each decade of a man's life until fifty, when it undergoes a drastic reduction in thickness of from six to eight microns each decade. I use this microscopic information only to demonstrate that aging makes each hair on our heads even more fragile and susceptible to banishment.

Although growth rate varies from man to man, it usually takes almost two and a half months for a man's hair to grow an inch. Normal hair growth averages only about one seventy-second of an inch per day, a statistic gleefully ignored by military commanders and pushy barbers. Just as aging causes each strand to grow thinner in diameter, the hair will also not grow as long with the passing of time. Unless the styles of the late 1960s return, this change from a thirty-six-inch potential to something shorter will probably pass unnoticed.

How the hair grows is the key information we need, especially an understanding that growth comes in cycles that vary from person to person and even from strand to strand. That makes it necessary to generalize a bit to explain the process. The medical terms for these cycles are the *anagen* stage and the *telogen* stage. In the anagen stage, the hair is in a growth cycle that can last anywhere between two to six years. In the telogen stage, the hair is in what could be described as a rest period that lasts for close to three months. Remember, not every strand of hair atop your head goes into a growth or rest period at the same time. Between 10 and 15 percent of your hair will be resting at one time, while the remaining 85 to 90 percent will be climbing outward at its one-seventy-second-of-an-inch daily pace.

A Hairy Comb Is Not All Bad

With the possible exception of Ed "Kookie" Byrnes of 77 *Sunset Strip* fame, most young men pay little attention to their combs after they've used them for their designed purpose. But once a man gets a bit older, he becomes painfully aware of the strands of fallen hair remaining among the teeth after he has used it. Relax! This particular evidence of falling hair does not necessarily mean that you are on the verge of baldness. It can be simple verification that your scalp is functioning normally. Healthy hair follicles and papillae can produce only one strand of hair at a time; the old must be discarded in order to make room for the new. The hair you find in your comb is probably in the telogen or resting phase of the growth cycle. The papilla is preparing to shoot up another to replace it—if you are not susceptible to male pattern or other disorders. It is normal for a man to lose as many as 100 individual strands of hair per day. Of course, this becomes more of a problem for men thirty-five and older because all of our biological processes begin to slow down with age. It takes older men longer to produce noticeable new hairs, and almost all men will have less hair as they age. On the other hand, bidding farewell to the old and welcoming the new gives us an opportunity to start over, to compensate for the abuse of the dear departed with an assurance of intensive care for the newborn.

> *Question*: I just celebrated my thirty-eighth birthday, and I never noticed any hair left in my comb until recently. Now there seems to be a lot of it. My dad isn't bald. Why am I suddenly losing hair?
>
> *Answer*: Probably because you just "celebrated" your thirty-eighth birthday. Chances are, the hair was there all along but you felt too secure in your youthfulness to worry about it.

The foregoing answer might seem a bit flippant, but there's more truth than frivolity in it. Actually, a man with a full head of hair at thirty-eight is unlikely to go bald. It's natural to worry, but there's a fool-proof way to set your mind at ease. A word of warning: the method is neither easy nor pleasant. Pick a weekend day when you have the time and deliberately count the hairs that remain in your comb over the course of a day. Then repeat the process once a week for several months. The total number of hairs you count that first day isn't important. What does matter is a sudden or steady increase in the number of fallen hairs over a period of time. If the count doesn't rise dramatically, you have nothing to worry about. If you see a definite progression in your hair loss, you should make an immediate appointment with a dermatologist.

Scalp and Hair Types

1. Normal
2. Oily
3. Dry

Your scalp and hair should fit into one of these three general types. If you have already tested yourself for skin type, you will have little difficulty identifying your scalp or hair type. Men with oily skin are likely to have oily scalp and hair, and so on. That is why I believe that hair care is a natural extension of skin care. Your new knowledge about proper skin care has already given you a head start on the basic do's and don'ts of intelligent hair care.

The Facts About Healthy Hair

There are too many variables about male hair for me to attempt to supply direct information about your own without a personal examination. But here's a case where you can do it yourself. You can determine if your hair is basically healthy. A professional hair analyst discovers the health of the whole by testing a single strand for stretch, curl, and smoothness. You can test your own hair at home, without the use of machines.

Home Stress Test

1. Pluck three full strands of hair from your head with a tweezer

from a top area where the coverage is fullest and longest. Don't worry—they'll grow in again.

2. Grasp the longest of the three strands with your fingers, and gradually attempt to stretch it, using slow and deliberate tension to avoid breaking it. It should stretch almost a fifth of its length if it is healthy.

3. Take a second strand and hold it tightly between the thumb and forefinger of your left hand. Catch the hair with the nails of the right thumb and forefinger, close to where it's being held with the left hand. We want to test for a different kind of elasticity by imitating women who can put a beautiful curl in package ribbon by using of a pair of scissors. Substituting fingernails for scissor edge, dig in and scrape them outward along the length of the hair and release. With luck, the hair should roll back into a fairly tight curl. Next, take the right thumb and forefinger and gently stretch it out again to its full length, hold for a few seconds, and release. Healthy hair will recoil into a curl. Hair that is weak will either stay straight or only partially curl.

4. The third strand test will rely on your sense of touch. The outer surface of a strand of healthy hair should feel smooth. Hold the hair with the thumb and forefinger of your left hand and run your right forefinger and thumb down its length toward the root end. If you feel roughness, it means that you have been mistreating your hair.

This is a simple at-home test that will give you an idea of the current condition of your hair. If you flunk all three portions of this test, especially if you are under the age of forty, it means you are already in trouble or surely heading in that direction. At the same time, if you have a relatively thick covering of hair and are under forty, you will have plenty of opportunity to correct the condition and make certain that the new growth has a long and healthy life.

> *Question*: I'm confused. You said that there is little basic difference between the skin of men and women. You also say that hair is a byproduct of the skin. If that's the case, why do men grow bald while women don't?

Answer: I also said, at one point, *"Vive la difference!"* In this case, it's definitely "la difference" that makes the difference.

Sad to say, medical science still doesn't know all it should about the problem of male baldness. Women do lose hair as they grow older, but it's rare that you see a bald woman. The one thing that gets general agreement among all the experts is that extreme male hair loss is directly related to our production of the male sex hormone androgen. They don't know why this is the case, but studies have proved the theory. Both men and women produce a bit of the hormones of the other sex, but not enough to cause baldness in women or the need for a man to wear a bra. You may detest the idea of baldness, but think of the alternative! In fact, one series of scientific experiments performed on eunuchs with healthy heads of hair demonstrated that nearly all of these unfortunate volunteers suffered startling hair loss and a tendency toward pattern baldness soon after they began a series of injections with male hormones. The choice is clear, almost as if the obstetrician had handed your parents a questionnaire inside the deliver room:

> *Parents:* *It's now time to decide the future of your son. You have three choices. Check one only.*
> *I prefer my son to have:*
> _____ *a good sex life*
> _____ *a high paying job*
> _____ *a bald head*

Obviously, our actual choices are considerably better than that. There is no reason you can't have a good sex life *and* a bald head, as verified by a large segment of the entire population, male and female. More importantly, it's becoming clearly evident that fewer of us are going to be doomed to go through life with a glistening, hairless head. No matter what your age or the current condition of your hair, you now have numerous alternatives.

The Facts About Serious Hair Loss

Blaming the production of androgen and the aging process for male baldness does nothing to explain the teenaged hairlines and hirsuteness of masculine septuagenarians like Ronald Reagan and Tip O'Neill. They make it tempting to point to the acquisition of political power as a possible cure-all—until you remember the shiny pates of such predecessors as Dwight Eisenhower and Sam Rayburn. Most men produce similar amounts of androgen and yet end up with very different amounts of hair during their lifetimes. Hereditary factors seem to be the chief culprits in serious male hair loss. *Alopecia simplex* (premature balding) and *alopecia senilis* (elderly balding) are nearly identical in appearance and are generally lumped together under the general heading of *male pattern baldness*. Look to your ancestors. A history of baldness—on either the paternal or maternal side of your family—makes you a possible candidate for pattern baldness at some point during your lifetime.

That statement is the hardest truth about the mystery of abnormal hair loss. But there are few truly unalterable conclusions to be reached about pattern balding, and there's no reason for you to start shopping for a toupee just because an ancient picture of your great-grandfather shows him with a high hairline. A history of baldness on either side of your family should encourage you to take every sensible precaution to begin preserving what you have, because there is no way of predicting exactly when your follicles might develop an adverse reaction to your production of testosterone.

The noticeable hair loss of male pattern baldness usually begins at both corners of the forehead. A formerly straight hairline will recede fairly rapidly at the corners until the man is left with something of a widow's peak that was not at all evident before. On the other hand, almost every man's normal hair loss will begin at the forehead and temples where the hair is usually thinnest. A very gradual rising of the hairline should not be construed as a sure sign of eventual baldness—unless it begins in the late teens or early twenties.

A man destined for male pattern baldness will next have a noticeable hair loss on the rear portion of the crown of his head. To make it more confusing, men who will never grow bald also experience a thinning of hair in this area. But real pattern baldness in a susceptible man will soon leave this portion of the scalp devoid of cover. Because the bald place resembles the area shaved by medieval monks, it is usually called the monk's spot. Often, if a man parts his hair on the side, he will notice a widening part line leading to the monk's spot.

Hair loss

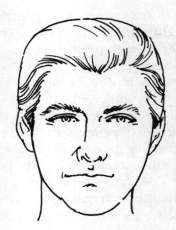

Normal twenties
hairline

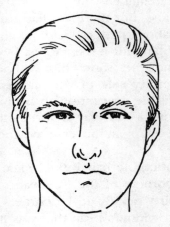

Normal twenties
hair loss

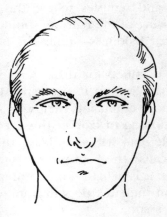

Twenties pattern
baldness

Hair loss

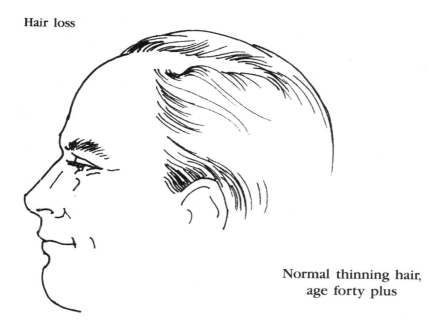

Normal thinning hair,
age forty plus

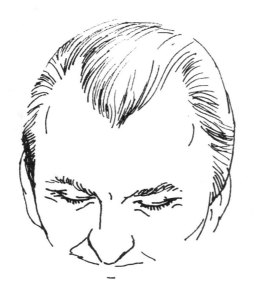

Male pattern baldness,
age twenty-five plus

Over the course of a very few years—and inherited male pattern baldness can begin as soon as the early twenties—the man with the unwanted legacy discovers that the hair on top of his head is continuing to grow thinner until his worst fears become reality. The sparse patches between his former hairline and the monk's spot disappear, and he is left with only a fringe around the sides and on the back of his head. This is the usual scenario for inherited pattern baldness. Most men will experience significant hair loss before they reach retirement age. However, they will retain enough to cut and comb. Even the tragedy of severe inherited baldness leaves many men with that healthy fringe of hair—and that gives them more than a ray of hope as, we shall see.

Inherited genes play a mystifying role in true male pattern baldness, and we have yet to come up with a fool-proof means of reversing the process for every man, but that is no reason to wave the white flag of surrender. The sooner the problem is attacked, the better our chances of lessening the damage. Age also plays an important part in the deterioration of men's hair, and that should act as another spur to get us working. The American Medical Association has released these figures which categorize the degree of noticeable baldness among American men:

Male Baldness

- Age 25   12%
- Age 35   37%
- Age 45   45%
- Age 65   65%

Statistics showing that the percentage of balding men grows in exact proportion to age at forty-five and beyond are exasperating in their tidiness. They create more frustration for a man in his twenties or early thirties who suffers from inherited baldness and must carry the stigma of this obvious sign of aging long before his time.

Other Causes of Abnormal Hair Loss

For the purposes of this book, let us assume you are still a youngish man—say, thirty-two years old—who can find absolutely no proof of a history of baldness on either side of his family. Yet you know that the number of loose hairs in your comb is growing by leaps and bounds. You know that some hair loss is completely normal. What's the problem? There are a number of other things that can cause us to lose abnormal amounts of hair. Knowing what they are can save us unnecessary worry—and hair.

General Ill Health

Poor health and some infectious diseases can wreak havoc on the hair. For that reason, if you notice a sudden unexplainable increase in hair loss it's wise to consult a doctor who can correct the problem that is affecting your overall health and your hair. Internal problems ranging from chronic constipation to hormonal imbalance to nervous disorders will sometimes first indicate their presence by their effect on the hair on our heads. Difficulties with the thyroid gland, for example, means that the body's metabolism will be affected and that can lead directly to a loss of hair. Any disease that brings on prolonged fevers can also trigger excessive hair loss, and, because the nervous system is biologically connected to the skin, any nervous disorder—even undue stress—can prompt skin problems as well as hair loss. The hair can act as a barometer of general health, and any unexplained loss of hair should encourage you to seek proper medical evaluation.

Dandruff, Infection, and Injury

Since it's even more prevalent than the common cold, dandruff is hardly considered a serious problem. Even some dermatologists view it more as an unsightly nuisance than a menace, but its ability to clog the pores and sebaceous glands of the scalp can make it a serious problem for anyone who is fighting pattern baldness. Dandruff, a form of seborrhoea, is another problem related to the production of our friendly nemesis sebum. Keeping the sebum produced by the scalp in proper balance is the best way to fight dandruff and the problems it presents in growing healthy hair. Sometimes, flaky and scaly scalp infections that we mistake for dandruff are really more serious problems that can actually cause bald patches. If your dandruff changes in appearance and doesn't improve with the better hygiene practices I will recommend, see a dermatologist. You could have ringworm or another fungus infection that could cause serious damage to your hair. The scalp is the manufacturing plant for your supply of hair, and anything in the way of injury—anything from excessive heat to traumatic wounds—can affect its normal operation and lead to excessive hair loss unless the condition is corrected.

Medications

Whether for medical or so-called recreational purposes, certain drugs can definitely be harmful to your hair. Amphetamines, even used under a doctor's guidance for other medical problems, can cause needless hair loss. So can thalium, anticoagulants, medicants containing arsenic, antithyroid drugs, anticancer drugs, and any preparations that contain sex hormones. Obviously, in a life-threatening situation such as cancer, the hair will have to take a back seat. But try to avoid a setback. Ask your physician how the prescribed drugs will affect your hair. Sometimes he or she can substitute one that will perform the same function without the harmful side effect.

Benign Neglect

I have saved this cause of hair loss for the end although it is not the least of the problem. Just as mismanagement of our daily approach to skin care can bring on all manner of problems and early aging, benign neglect of the hair is a sure way to ensure its early departure. Improper cleaning, the use of harmful products on the hair and scalp, the sun, excess heat, and environmental pollutants all contribute to early thinning and eventual hair loss.

Hair Loss—Quick Menu

1. Hair care is a natural extension of informed skin care.
2. Blond men are originally endowed with more hair follicles than brunets, while redheads have fewer but thicker individual hairs.
3. Visible hair is dead material, 97 percent protein, composed of three layers.

4. The loss of sixty to a hundred individual strands of hair per day is normal as hair goes from the anagen to telogen stage.

5. Men suffer more hair loss than women because of the yet unexplained working of the male sex hormones.

6. Heredity is the greatest cause of pattern baldness in men.

7. A history of baldness on either the father or mother's side of the family can make any man a likely candidate for inherited baldness.

8. Noticeable hair loss increases with age until 65 percent of American men aged sixty-five will have varying degrees of baldness.

9. General ill health—impaired blood circulation, hormonal imbalance, glandular and nervous disorders—can prompt abnormal hair loss.

10. Dandruff and other scalp infections can result in bald patches.

11. Scalp injury, prolonged fevers, and lesser traumas can lead to unnecessary hair loss.

9

Fighting Back: Defenses Against Hair Loss

It is clear that noticeable hair loss is a mysterious and complex condition that will trouble the majority of all men at some point in their lifetimes. Early recognition of the potential problem will give you a head start in the battle to keep your hair. Everyone wants a magic pill that will immediately end fallout, grow hair, and restore color to its teenage glory. It has not been invented. Until it is, we must rely on hard work and common sense to get the job done.

> *Question*: I'm very concerned about shampooing. I used to wash my hair almost every morning until about a year ago when I noticed the drain was getting clogged with the hair I was trying to clean. Does too much shampooing cause baldness?

There was a time when it was widely believed that washing the hair too often could cause baldness. The opposite is true. A sound program of hygiene is vital—as with the face—to keep the pores and oil ducts of your scalp open and functioning. This encourages the healthy growth of hair. However, depending on your skin and hair type, too much washing with the wrong kind of product can affect the hair's normal growing and resting phases. Most men, depending on their work and leisure activities, have no real need for a daily shampoo. Generally speaking, the rules that apply for cleaning your skin type—normal, dry, or oily—will also work best for your hair and scalp because they will have inherited the same tendencies.

Oily Hair

The sebaceous glands of both face and scalp are working overtime to cause the greasy, stuck-together look of your hair. Therefore, it is important that you shampoo more often for both the appearance and the health of your hair and scalp. You should not forget that the oil glands have a tendency to increase production to offset your attempt to slow them down. Unnecessary washing with an overly strong shampoo could prove to be counterproductive. Experiment until you find the right combination. Use a mild shampoo for oily hair, and try washing it every other day.

Dry Hair

Dry hair is usually bred by dry skin and is caused by the same problem: an insufficient amount of sebum. The natural oil must make its way up the hair shaft to keep it supple. Dry hair is especially brittle, from follicle to the end, and must be treated very carefully. It is usually more inclined to break and split and is also less capable of maintaining its hold on the scalp. The fortunate thing about dry hair is that it has less tendency to collect dirt. For that reason it doesn't need as many thorough cleanings. A man with dry hair should use a mild shampoo formulated for his type and rich in protein. Under normal circumstances, dry hair does not need to be washed more than three times a week. Find what works best for you.

Normal Hair

A man with so-called normal hair probably has perfect skin as well. He should first thank God for his good fortune, then his mother and father. Shampoo as frequently as you feel the need, using a product that is not harsh, and make certain that you don't change the balance of nature by abusing the hair with foreign substances that will claim to make it look better.

Rule: Never use your bath or face soap to shampoo your hair.

There's a natural tendency for any busy man to climb into his morning shower, realize that he still has time to wash his hair, and remember that the shampoo is on a shelf across the bathroom. Do not take the easy way out and lather your scalp and hair with your bath soap. I would prefer that you use your special face soap on your entire body. Skin, after all, is skin. I certainly disapprove of using face or bath soap on such a sensitive area as your scalp and hair. The soap ingredients of fat and lye can commit murder on your hair.

Question: My hair is definitely thinning, and my wife says I should use baby shampoo, claiming that anything safe for a baby has to be okay for an adult. What's your feeling?

The reasoning sounds sensible, but there's a fly in the ointment or, more accurately, a flaw in the shampoo. Most baby shampoos are as gentle as a young child's hair is tough, but the primary gentleness comes from additives designed to keep the mixture from stinging baby's eyes during the washing. This works fine for little children, but those same chemicals can have an adverse reaction on the super-sensitive hair follicles of an adult male. I would stay away from baby shampoo.

Although they've invented no curative for hair loss that works for everyone, manufacturers have done an excellent job in formulating men's shampoos that are safe and efficient. Even if you have oily hair, it's best to use a shampoo that is more acidic than alkaline. An alkaline cleaner can wreak havoc with the hard outer surface of the hair and destroy the cuticle's protective armor. For that reason, avoid all detergent-based and other harsh shampoos. The milder acidic shampoos will help lock moisture inside the hair and make for a more lustrous look. Remember, too, that hair is 97 percent protein and some of that protein will be washed away with each shampoo. That's why I prefer a shampoo that contains protein. The hair manages to absorb some of it to make up for that lost in the cleaning. These are general guidelines in selecting a shampoo.

Problem hair can be even more fragile than troublesome skin, and selecting a shampoo that will clean without harming your hair is your first order of business.

The old idea of getting hair squeaky clean is not really sensible. Your goal is to keep both the hair and the scalp clean without robbing either of its natural moisture. Educated shampooing is as important to the life of your hair as proper shaving is to the appearance of your face. The following program may seem boringly elementary, but it is vitally important in helping you make the most of what you've got.

Sensible Shampooing

1. Select a mild, nondetergent shampoo suitable for your individual hair type—oily, dry, or normal.

2. Men with excessively oily or normal hair can shampoo as needed, probably every other day. Men with dry hair should limit their shampoos to three a week or fewer.

3. A shower, using warm rather than hot water, after your morning skin care routine is the best place and time for a shampoo. A shower offers maximum soaking and rinsing.

4. Soak the hair thoroughly, pour an adequate amount of shampoo into the palm of your hand, dilute with a bit of water, and begin to work into a lather.

5. Apply lather to sides and top of the head, using more water to increase lather, and massage gently through the hair and over the scalp, using the fingertips.

6. One lathering per shampoo should be enough to clean hair and scalp.

7. Rinse very thoroughly to make certain no residue is left on the scalp or individual strands of hair.

8. If time permits, gently pat dry with a towel.

Chances are, you are already shampooing in this manner. But, as in shaving, it's tough to break harmful routines learned early—such as using water that's overly hot—and it's tempting to get lackadaisical in the interest of saving time. As we age, the hair on our heads becomes more precious and deserving of our full attention. Sensible shampooing is exactly what it says, a good first step in avoiding calamitous hair loss.

Question: Is there any truth in the story that regular, vigorous massage of the scalp will produce new hair?

As they said in the 1960s, "If it feels good, do it!" With that preface, let me add that there is no scientific evidence that vigorous massage will help the growth of hair. I am in favor of gentle massage for the scalp during the course of the regular shampoo because all massage is relaxing and will help stimulate the circulation of blood. The hair follicles in the dermis of the scalp need a good blood supply to remain healthy, but there is no reason to expect a sudden resurgence of hair growth because of massage. Any hair manipulation should be gentle to avoid damage that might not be correctable. Too many men forget this while shampooing and traumatize their scalps by digging in with their fingernails. Cease and desist this practice.

Question: What is this business about towel drying your hair? Mine is getting pretty thin on top, but I can make it looker fuller and younger by styling it while I dry it with a hair blower. It's also faster. Is there anything wrong with a man's hair dryer?

I must give you a qualified answer on this one: not if it is used with care. The blow-gun hair dryer so popular with men is near and dear to my heart, in part because of its symbolism. When the portable hair blower made its unabashed and unexpected appearance in the locker rooms of professional sports teams a few years back, it encouraged a wide spectrum of the male population to acknowledge that there was nothing "sissy" about a desire to improve their personal grooming and appearance. That was a real breakthrough for men. These dryers are extremely practical aids for a man on a busy schedule, and they really can help make a head of thinning hair look fuller.

A strong word of caution is necessary: excessive heat is potentially harmful both to the scalp and to the hair that is growing from it. Women, who have flowing manes seldom affected by real pattern baldness, can get away with using the deluxe models that throw out plenty of super-heated air. Men must be more careful. A man who wants to preserve his hair should always avoid using a dryer at maximum heat. It's advisable to hold the dryer from eight to twelve inches away from the hair to be dried, and you might even experiment with the dryer on its lowest heat cycle. For that matter, there's a wide selection of dryers on the market, and it's eminently sensible to shop for one that caters specifically to your needs, one that operates on low wattage and puts an automatic governor on the accelerator, lest you forget and get carried away.

> *Question*: I can remember my grandmother telling my
> sister something about 100 strokes a day with
> a brush being good for the hair. Is brushing
> that much good for a man's hair too?

That's another of the old wives' tales that has pretty much fallen by the wayside, especially for men. Of course, women adhering to that dictum have never had as much to lose. Too much brushing can be detrimental to a man's hair. The original idea was to spread the natural oils and moisturizers of the scalp throughout the hair and make it more lustrous. That was fine as far as it went. But if you're worried about thinning hair, you know that a rugged session with a hair brush can create more panic than you used to feel when your father approached with the same instrument, intent on applying its reverse side to your backside. Vigorous brushing will attack weakened hair like a lawn rake cleaning out a yard full of autumn leaves. I don't think the temporary benefits are worth the long-term risk.

Another form of hair loss, usually associated with women, is one that medical science calls *traction alopecia*. In layman's language, it refers to healthy hair that is gradually pulled from the scalp by external pressure. Most women bring on the problem by pulling the hair back tightly and holding it in a rubber band or similar device to fashion a bun or ponytail. Men can develop the same problem by putting any excess stress on the hair, even through overly strong brushing and rough combing. Once past your third decade, you will have less ability to regrow hair lost through traction. Occasional gentle brushing of the hair can be therapeutic, but it's best to use a good natural-bristle brush. Fine-toothed plastic combs with needlelike teeth can also be damaging to the scalp if used constantly. Anything that puts almost constant pressure on your scalp and hair—from crash helmets to overly tight hats or caps to elastic sweatbands to crowns—can speed up the natural process of thinning hair.

Rules: **1.** Never let Hulk Hogan grab you by the hair and throw you around a "rassling ring."
2. Never use a fine-toothed comb or brush to style thoroughly wet hair.

These rules are simply intended to remind you of the obvious. Anything that puts undue tension on that valuable stuff on top of your head is a capital-letter DON'T. Let common sense be your guide.

Question: I'm thirty-three, I have a full head of hair, and I don't think I'll ever be bald. But I can bend over and comb or brush my hair forward and make the space around my head look like a January blizzard in Buffalo. I've tried, but I can't seem to get rid of dandruff. Do you have any fool-proof suggestions?

Only one: if it's as bad as you say, take your problem to a good dermatologist. Even a doctor may not be able to help because common dandruff is something that continues to mystify or escape the attention of the medical profession. However, a doctor can tell you if the problem is anything more serious than dandruff and give you treatment for it. The simplest way of controlling a dandruff problem is by frequent shampooing, especially if you have oily or normal hair. Most dandruff is caused by overactive sebaceous glands combined with the normal scaling and shedding of the scalp's epidermis.

Here again, the industry that makes grooming aids has come up with some pretty reliable products to help us. If you have dandruff that's embarrassing or potentially damaging to your hair, try one of the antidandruff shampoos on the market. Most of them contain such additives as selenium pyrithione, zinc, sulfur, salycylic acid, or tar. They can be very effective in keeping most dandruff under control. Try one for a couple of weeks, and if you're not pleased with the results, keep shopping until you find one that does the job for you.

Let me tell you a story that set me testing a commercial product with a pretty dismal name that is as old as the proverbial hills. On one of my appearances on the Merv Griffin show, I was discussing skin and hair care, and Merv mentioned that he had been worried as a young man about falling hair. He tried an old product called Glover's Mange Cure and found that it really worked for him. His unpaid testimonial before millions on national television was verified by the head of healthy hair he has today. Glover's might also work for you, although each individual's scalp and hair are different. You might be surprised that I have suggested that numerous patients with threatening dandruff try the Glover's Mange Cure created for veterinarians to use on the coats of animals. This is a heavy-duty product that can get marvelous results for humans. Needless to say, I would advise any individual to first consult a dermatologist to make certain this or any other special product was entirely safe and suitable for his particular use.

> *Question*: I see that companies are now putting out hair conditioners for men. I know women have used them for years. Do they do any good?

They're not going to grow hair or even bring natural hair loss to a screeching halt, but I would say they are worthwhile for any man who wants to keep his thinning hair in the best shape. Conditioners that contain protein can be especially useful for men with dry, thinning hair. A good protein conditioner will help seal the moisture inside each hair on the head and help alleviate the worst effects of the problem. Basically, conditioners make the hair easier to manage and a less likely subject for unintentional tension damage from combing or brushing. The grooming industry has yet to come up with a single product that will make every man's hair perfect, but I'm a firm believer in shopping around to take advantage of new technology that can make hair care safer and simpler. Read the labels, follow the directions, and give it a shot.

> *Question*: Are hair thickeners, sprays, mousses, and other dressings effective? Are they dangerous to use on a man's hair?

I'll give that question a yes-and-no answer, with a qualifying "depending on the individual." First, let's tackle the problem of possible danger. Most of these products do contain varying amounts of alcohol, and too much of that substance can be drying. On the other hand, the companies who manufacture the products cannot afford to sell you something that will cause you to lose your hair. If you follow the directions and pay close attention to the results, the danger of any of these commercial aids seriously damaging your hair is minimal. Sprays, mousses, and thickeners do add control and an appearance of more hair for many men. The so-called dry look was a decided boon for men with thinning hair. Using the new dry, soft-hold applications in combination with some clever combing can make a man's hair look much fuller. Unfortunately, none of these products can do much for a man with ultra-sparse, dry hair on the crown of his head. That man would be best advised to skip all hair dressings, save a protein shampoo. The wet look has been making something of a comeback in men's hair styling in recent years. This style is not at all beneficial for a man with aged or thinning hair, because the clumping effect of the oily dressing only makes him seem to have less hair. The one hair dressing I strongly oppose is the brilliantine type that is heavily oil based. Adding more oil to a scalp that produces adequate amounts is only asking for trouble, and it's almost certain to follow if used by a man who has hair that's already too oily.

> *Question*: I work for a very conservative Wall Street firm, and I guess I'm pretty straightforward when it comes to my haircuts. My hair used to be very thick, but it's gotten alarmingly thin on top over the past five years. Is it true a man's hair stylist can cut it in a way to make it look fuller?

Absolutely! Of course, no stylist can work miracles for a man with very little hair. My field of expertise is in the inner working of the skin and hair, and I make no claims about hair cutting or styling. But logic dictates that it's possible to cut, style, and even comb thinning hair in a way that will enhance what's there. Finding an expert hair cutter, whether he or she is called a barber or a hair stylist, is an important step for a man with thinning hair. The person who does the job should also be someone who will listen to what you say. Anyone who brags that he or she knows many different hair styles is about as useful as a shoemaker who can make numerous styles of shoes in sizes from one to six. If you wear a size ten, who needs him? Never hesitate to tell the barber what you expect to achieve from your haircut. After all, it's your head and your hair. If he or she can't do the job, find another barber.

At the same time, there's a point of diminishing returns in attempting to cover an extensively bald pate by outlandish cuts or styles. If you allow the hair right above your ears to grow abnormally long and sweep it low across your forehead or drape it across a bare crown hoping to disguise widespread loss of hair, the resultant strange hairline, part, and overall "do" are more likely simply to call attention to your problem. Doing the best you can is the name of this game, and, although eventual baldness is a depressing subject, there are many options on the way.

> *Question*: I'm thankful that I have plenty of hair, but some of it started to turn gray at the age of eighteen. I'm now twenty-eight and the gray streaks are really getting noticeable. I'm in a very competitive career where the emphasis seems to be on youth. Is there any way to color hair that's both safe and subtle?

This is one of the happiest areas of hair care to talk about because men have also "come a long way, baby" in returning their hair to its youthful shade. Hair-coloring products in general have been steadily improved over the years to make them simple to apply, natural-looking, and safe for the hair and scalp, providing you use the suggested patch test or check with a dermatologist to make certain you will have no adverse reaction.

Why We Turn Gray

Graying, like baldness, is related to both the aging process and hereditary factors. Heredity will cause a few men to begin turning gray very early in adulthood, most men will have a hard time counting every gray hair on their heads by the time they reach their forties, and some men with lucky genes never seem to gray or lose hair. In rare instances, a vitamin deficiency can cause unnatural graying, and this can be helped by treatment with a B vitamin called para-aminobenzoic acid. However, there is no medical treatment that can reverse graying in every man. It has also been proved that extreme stress can cause some men to turn gray "before their time." Thus, the old legend about a young soldier becoming white-haired overnight in the heat of combat is not without some truth. But in most cases, your ancestors and date of birth are the principal malefactors.

How We Can Get Rid of the Gray

With all of the fine products on the market today, there is just no reason for any man with premature gray hair to let it bother him. Even older men who have career or personal reasons for wanting to look younger should not allow the lack of pigment in their hair to slow them down. Many older celebrities in recent years have opted for the natural look and allowed the gray to show after years of touch-ups, but if gray hair is a concern to you, get rid of it.

If you have the time and money, going to a hair professional is undoubtedly the easiest and best way of returning your hair to its youthful coloring. On the other hand, doing it yourself is not really that difficult. Many men particularly approve of the so-called color restorers that gradually return color to something close to its original shade. Others find that some of these substances work too slowly and sometimes give them a rather orangish tint. In my practice I have found, perhaps surprisingly, that a majority of men find the most satisfactory coloring aid one that is not even advertised to appeal to men. These men swear by Clairol's Loving Care, a longtime favorite of their wives and sweethearts. They like the simple directions and easy application and feel confident that the finished job looks completely natural. A decided plus is the fact that any dissatisfaction can be effectively shampooed away in less than two weeks. On that subject, I feel it's far safer to go with a coloring product that is clearly temporary rather than a permanent dye.

Words of Caution

If your youthful hair color could be best described as black, never try to color it back to its original shade. A black hair color, regardless of the manufacturer's claims, will leave men looking as if they had soaked their heads in black liquid shoe polish. Naturally black hair has so many variations in shade that it is virtually impossible to duplicate. Age causes subtle changes in complexion color that intensify the unnatural look of jet black hair, and it's wiser to experiment with deep shades of brown. Advance testing can save embarrassment and time. Ask your barber to save some large clumps of your cut hair during your next visit. Take these home and try different shades on them before you try it on the hair that's intact. That way, you'll know exactly what you're going to get.

Miracle Cures That Could Correct Your Baldness

Our hair care program, to this point, has centered on the best possible methods of preserving, protecting, and enhancing the youthful good looks of the growing hair on a man's head. But what about the man who knows he's already beyond normal hair care, the man who knows he's facing the prospect of real baldness?

It requires neither super intelligence nor some deep-seated cynicism about high-flown advertising claims to recognize that my sensational headline actually hedges its bet. Fair enough. It was honestly intended to do that. The operative word in that headline is *could.* The problem with ads for most so-called miracle cures for baldness is that they claim the product being sold *will* cure baldness. There is, to the best of anyone's knowledge, no product that can honestly make that blanket claim.

As I have already said, it is impossible to grow hair on a billiard ball, and it is at this time equally impossible to grow new hair on a man with a scalp that has been cue-ball smooth for twenty years. Those are the sad facts. On the other hand, there are methods and products that have succeeded in stimulating hair growth on men with new baldness. None of these products have been universally approved by the Federal Drug Administration or the medical establishment in America as sure cures for pattern baldness. The scientific community works very slowly, as we all know, in testing every possible effect of a new drug or substance before giving it an official stamp of approval. This is a highly commendable aim because get-rich-quick operators have already raised false hopes and made vast fortunes in schemes to sell "miracle" products to those afflicted with incurable physiological problems. Certainly, since the beginning of recorded history, people have made money peddling cures for baldness.

But the well-intentioned caution of the scientific community does nothing to relieve the anxiety of a man who would do almost anything to see the return of a bit of hair to the top of his head. I believe some guarded optimism is now justified. I am encouraged because I have seen the evidence with my own eyes. What follows is not a personal endorsement of the substances I am going to mention. By all means, get a dermatologist's advice about your own chances of success before you spend time and money investing in a possible cure. Never forget that none of these products will work for everyone. My intention in setting down this information is purely journalistic. These methods have been helpful in correcting pattern baldness in some men. You might be among the lucky ones.

Minoxidil

This drug was first produced by the Upjohn Pharmaceutical Company as a scientifically proven aid in controlling high blood pressure. It was fully tested and approved for this purpose by the FDA and the medical establishment. Its potential as a hair grower came about by sheer accident. Some of the patients who were using the drug to fight high blood pressure suddenly noticed that they were growing excess amounts of hair, often on the face, wrists, and other places where they had no need for it. When they complained of this curious side effect of Minoxidil, Upjohn scientists began experimenting on the possible use of the drug in solution form as a means of growing hair on the bald spots of the head. Meticulous tests were conducted in several centers across the nation, with the eager subjects applying the Minoxidil solution to their bald spots morning and night for several months. The tests proved to the satisfaction of the Upjohn researchers that the Minoxidil solution did actually grow new hair on some people. Of the 2,000 tested in the original go-round, about one-third reported some new hair growth.

The testing of Minoxidil to this point indicates that men who have developed bald spots on the crowns of their heads within the past five years have the best chance of benefiting from its use. The drug is far less successful in correcting the baldness associated with a receding hairline, and there seems to be little if any benefit for men who have had overall baldness for a long period of time. The tests also indicated that the Minoxidil solution slows the process of hair loss in men who have not yet gone completely bald. But this is no perfect solution, no matter how you look at it. Applications must be continued indefinitely or the new hair will fall out, and a

Minoxidil solution, whether the product put out by Upjohn or a lotion concocted by your local pharmacist, is very costly. Regular daily applications may cost you many hundreds of dollars each year, and you can multiply that to thousands over the course of a life-time. Are the results worth that kind of expenditure? You must continue using it to get satisfactory results.

The FDA has not yet approved the Minoxidil solution as a safe and effective method of growing hair. However, the drug has been cleared by the FDA for use against high blood pressure, and its sale is not illegal. FDA spokesmen say they are worried about possible side effects for men who use it as a hair restorer but have no history of high blood pressure. Using it externally can cause some of the powerful drug to be absorbed into the system where it can create problems. For that reason, you must get the advice of your doctor before you attempt to use it.

The bottom line is that it is available, it is legal, and it has worked for some men. There is no evidence that it has created a thick, flowing head of hair for anyone. Expectations should not be too high, even if you fit into the category of those it has helped. This seems a likely place to mention that another such drug used to control high blood pressure—Diazoxide—also has a side effect of hirsutism. It is not as well known as Minoxidil, but some men have also credited it with growing hair on bald spots. If you have the money, the patience, and the motivation, it might be worth your while to learn more about these still experimental curatives for lost hair.

Banfi

This is a commercial product manufactured in Hungary that created an unprecedented demand when it was introduced in Europe more than fifteen years ago and a storm of controversy when it later attempted to gain entry into the United States. It was emphatically denied the seal of approval of the Federal Drug Administration and is illegal in the United States. I include it here, not to defy the FDA, but only because a number of my European clients have used it and swear by it. Presumably, if you want to try it, you'll have to arrange for a European friend to buy it or journey there yourself and bring it back with you.

Banfi backs its claims with official documentation from the Medical University Hospital of Budapest. That Hungarian report says that Banfi was scientifically tested there on forty men and women in 1980, and the final results were most impressive. According to the report, none of those tested was unchanged at the end, 66 percent were improved, and 34 percent were considered recovered. The report explains that "improved" meant that hair loss had been reduced or partial hair growth had been identified in formerly bald spots. "Recovered" meant that "loss of hair had ceased, or almost ceased, or had been reduced to a minimum." The Budapest report also claimed that the hair lotion had no side effects in the cases examined.

Obviously, any American who wants to use this product has a choice that echoes the world political situation. Whom do you trust, the American Federal Drug Administration or the Communist Hungarian medical people? The FDA says the Budapest testing was not up to American standards, but millions of men on the continent and in England have paid over thirty dollars for a bottle that will last them from eight to ten weeks. The normal length of their hair growth course is advertised to last between three and six months.

Products That Claim to Stop Hair Loss

There are a number of products that stop short of claiming success in growing new hair on balding heads but insist that they are capable of arresting the loss of falling hair. I will list the three that have records of the best success. Interestingly, all of these products have beeen cleared by the FDA and are sold in the United States.

Bioscal. The approach here is as a preventive treatment for the scalp, with claims of success in stopping excessive hair loss, flaky dandruff, oil imbalances, and itchiness. Recommended treatment with the Bioscal preparation is on a daily basis for a period of six or seven months. That can be expensive.

Physicians Products Progesterone Hair System. This treatment works on the theory that Dihydrotestosterone (DHT) is the specific hormone responsible for male pattern baldness and is designed to counteract its harmful reaction on a man's hair. The manufacturer says that progesterone safely reduces the production of DHT from testosterone and thus helps in stopping excessive hair loss. This also is no nonprofit corporation.

Physicians Clinics Scalp Care System. This company supplies another lotion that utilizes progesterone to "suppress the conversion of testosterone to dihydrotestosterone" and supposedly end hair loss. It is not available in stores but does not need a doctor's prescription and can be ordered direct from the company. A one-month supply (eight ounces) comes in at a price tag near twenty-five dollars.

As you can see, there's no lack of activity in the search for a miracle cure for baldness or even some medication that can arrest abnormal hair loss that has begun. I can make no blanket endorsement for any of these products except to say that some of them have been helpful to some men. Obviously, the sooner you attack the problem of insipient baldness, the better your chances for success. It certainly helps to have unlimited money and lucky genes.

Surgery: A Proven Alternative

By far the most tested and successful way of getting some of your own hair growing back on top of your head is with the aid of the tools of a plastic surgeon. Frank Sinatra, Hugh Downs, Senator William Proxmire, and scores of other famous men have undergone hair operations of some kind and have had successful results. There is no doubt at all that surgical procedures to move hair from one part of the head to another do work. The problem is that they do not work for all men.

You are not a good candidate for hair transplanting if you have too little or no hair at all somewhere on your scalp. A healthy fringe of hair above the ears and at the back of the head is a must. Hereditary traits figure vitally even in surgical procedures because you must have a family background of persistently healthy hair on the lower portions of the scalp, even if everyone in your family's past sported a bald top. Not all of the bald areas of ideal candidates, particularly the forehead, are always receptive to transplants. Above all, the hair to be transplanted must come from follicles that are certain to remain normally productive for the rest of your life. If all of these criteria are met, you will have your own healthy hair sprouting on a formerly bare or thinning patch within three months. There are several methods of transferring your own hair from a thickly populated area to a bald or thinning spot.

Hair Plug Transplants

This form of surgical hair transplanting has been in general use since 1959. It is a relatively simple procedure that can be performed in the doctor's office under mild sedation or novocaine. Once the doctor verifies that your chances for success are good, he or she will use a punch-type device that will lift small patches of follicles, skin, and hair from the back or sides of your head. The perfect plugs, less than a sixth of an inch in diameter, will contain a number of healthy hair follicles that can be counted on to grow in the selected and prepared new site. Anywhere from twenty-five to one hundred plugs can be moved at each session with the surgeon. The number of visits you will need depends on the extent of scalp you want to cover and the availability of your transplantable hair.

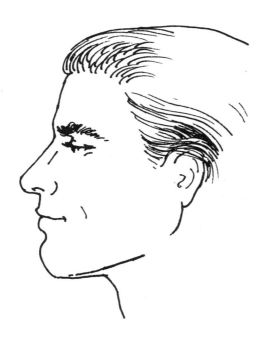

Hair plugs

The plugs are usually secured in the new area by pressure at the time of implantation, although stitches are sometimes used to cut down on bleeding and excess scarring. Like most kinds of plastic surgery, the costs will vary from surgeon to surgeon. Generally, you can expect to pay about fifteen dollars per hair plug. That means you must be prepared to fork over close to $3,000 to beef up a bit of thinning to more than $6,000 to cover up some wide-open spaces. There's almost no way to keep the operation a secret from the folks at the office because the results are necessarily notice-able, transplant sessions are usually separated by six-week intervals, the transplanted hair quickly falls out before the new growth be-comes visible in three months or so, and it will probably take at least ten months before you get the full growth of hair you dreamed of. Still, this is *the* time-tested way of growing your own hair if you are biologically suitable and financially solvent.

Scalp Reduction and Scalp-Flap Procedures

These are newer and, according to some, more efficient and basi-cally safer techniques of transferring growing hair from one area of the scalp to another. Scalp reduction is an operation that does pretty much what the name implies. In a manner similar to that used in a face lift, incisions are made which allow the surgeon to cut away bald areas of the scalp and replace them with the adjacent skin that contains healthy hair. The scalp-flap surgery is more com-plicated and is best suited for a man whose most troublesome hair loss is at the front of the head. In this procedure, healthy strips of hair-growing tissue, as long as five inches, are surgically removed from above each of the ears and transplanted so that they join above the forehead. According to those who favor this technique, the transplanted hair is less prone to instant fallout and slow re-growth as in hair plug transplants. However, in both scalp-flap and the similar strip graft transplant, hair plugs are often used to make the new hairline look more natural. Depending on the amount of hair being moved, the more complicated nature of these operations can make them even more expensive than hair plug transfers. Their potential, especially in helping men with receding hairlines, is an-other great leap forward in the battle against baldness.

If you are seriously contemplating further investigation into the possibility of a hair transplant, it is extremely important that you remember two things, even if you are a viable candidate for such procedures: (1) this plastic surgery is going to cost you more than just a few bucks and, (2) it's a long process that will take almost a year before you begin to feel that you got your money's worth.

When All Else Fails

Toupees

The dictionary defines it as "a small wig or section of false hair worn to cover a bald spot." Too many men faced with the need of buying a toupee might consider it "a preliminary death shroud, used to cover a naked scalp while one is still alive." There's no argument that baldness without hope is a deeply disturbing problem. It is a predicament that requires careful self-analysis and a weighing of available options. The ability to accept what is happening and to know that it has no reflection whatsoever on your worth as a man is a visible display of character. If the baldness fills you with uncontrollable insecurity and self-doubt, you can still put yourself back in the driver's seat. Buy a hair piece.

Without ever having discussed the matter with him personally, I feel that producer–director–actor–comedian Carl Reiner has the healthiest public attitude imaginable about his own baldness. Carl developed baldness early in life and freely admits to owning dozens of hair pieces in various styles. Yet he wears one in public only if his profession demands it, or because he simply feels in the mood to do so. To be or not to be (bald, that is) is a decision that gives him little evident anxiety. Actors who have suffered the worries of early male pattern baldness have not let it deter their careers or their obvious sex appeal. Ask your women friends if the fact that Burt Reynolds wears a toupee interferes with his macho image.

It's the memory of the old-fashioned bad toupee—the proverbial "rug"—that causes men to shudder when they contemplate wearing one. Fortunately, the art of making hair pieces has progressed at a pace worthy of science that tries to make them obsolete. You can now purchase a custom-made hair piece—tiny or large—that is natural-looking and virtually undetectable. The fuller styles of normal hair plus careful fitting and ingenious blending with your own hair heighten the naturalness of today's finest toupees. It takes about a month—from first visit when a toupee maker measures your head, makes a mold to ensure a perfect fit, and helps you select the proper color—before you can first don your new hair. You can expect to pay $1,000 or more for a really fine hairpiece, and you will be told you must give it almost as much care as you would your own growing hair. For that reason—toupees must be kept clean—a man who is serious about projecting a natural appearance would find it advantageous to buy more than one piece. Thus, even this not altogether satisfying means of having hair is going to cost real money. Still, the cost is little if your insecurity about baldness is great.

Other Options

A technique generally categorized as hair weaving (despite a tendency of some companies to give it a more substantial-sounding label) is favored by many men who are not yet bald but who have extensive loss of hair. The upbeat psychological effect of this beefing-up process of natural hair is probably its best benefit. The original effect is wonderfully satisfying if done properly. Unfortunately, it can be nothing but a temporary satisfaction because new, matching human hair is only attached to the hair that already exists. That means constant revisions are necessary as the growing hair falls out. This kind of replacement technique can actually be twice as expensive as purchasing a toupee, and the necessary repeat visits for new adjustments can cost an additional $300 or more per year. That seems to me a poor investment.

> *Rule*: Never subject yourself to the danger inherent in a supposedly permanent artificial hair replacement called surgical implant.

Because I greatly empathize with any man who suffers from baldness, I am generally in favor of trying almost anything that will enable him to look better and gain confidence. However, the process labeled surgical implant is not one I can endorse. The original idea—to take hair that a man cannot grow himself and surgically attach it to the scalp so he never has to remove it—seemed almost too good to be true. It was! Surgical implants became popular a few years ago until dangerous complications grew out of the procedure. Many men developed very serious infections arising from the surgery, and even a few deaths resulted. Fortunately, most of the clinics have now gone out of business. A few remain to entice the unwary. I consider this technique highly dangerous and one to be avoided.

If you have thoroughly digested everything in this section on hair care, you should appreciate the fact that total understanding of a man's hair is a mystery that the entire scientific community will be unable to unravel until some time in the future. The most obvious fact about preserving your own hair is that proper care cannot begin too early, whatever the nature of your family history. Just how truly precious is this keratinized substance that grows—or once grew—on our heads? Only you can really make that judgment call. Hair loss resulting from improper care and poor information is a battle we can fight and win.

Fighting Back—Quick Menu

1. Frequent shampooing is more likely to prevent rather than cause excessive hair loss.

2. Never use a face or bath soap to shampoo your hair.

3. Use a gentle acidic shampoo suitable for your hair type.

4. Shampoo in warm rather than hot water, and lather only once.

5. Repeated massage that is too vigorous can do more harm than good.

6. Excessive heat from hair dryers is potentially dangerous.

7. Strong combing or brushing of wet hair or anything that exerts unusual pressure on the hair and scalp can cause hair loss.

8. Dependable treatments are available to control dandruff.

9. Conditioners, thickeners, sprays, and other dressings are generally safe and can make a man's hair appear fuller.

10. Choose your barber carefully, he or she can help you make the most of the hair you have.

11. There are no medical cures for most graying, but home coloring is generally safe, simple, and natural-looking.

12. Never attempt to color hair black. The result seldom looks natural.

13. New drugs are available that have proved effective in growing new hair on the heads of some men.

14. Other recent nonprescription products have demonstrated some success in stopping abnormal hair loss.

15. Surgical procedures—hair plug, scalp reduction, and scalp-flap transplants—have a history of proven effectiveness in transferring a man's own hair from one area on his scalp to another.

16. Improved, undetectable toupees and hair pieces make baldness a personal choice instead of a possible embarrassment.

10

What's on the Market

Because I have no personal axe to grind, I have—with only a few exceptions—carefully avoided making recommendations of name brand grooming products throughout the pages of this book. However, I have no desire to put you at a disadvantage in finding the products that will work best in your personal skin and hair care program. This chapter may open up a world of new possibilities to you.

Most men, accustomed to doing their toiletries shopping at the nearest supermarket, simply have no idea of the enormous range of products recently developed specifically for men. The fact that so many famous old companies have now created entire lines of products especially for men should add substance to your decision to take better care of your skin and hair. You are now a member of one of the fastest-growing men's clubs in existence. On the lists that follow, you will be able to find name-brand examples of all the various products, suitable for your type skin and hair, that have been discussed in this book.

I have purposely not included prices for the products listed, but it's wise to remember—the bigger the name, the bigger the cost. Also, a higher price does not always assure you of a more effective product. All of the companies listed also produce such standard products as colognes, after-shave lotions, shave foams, and other items I have not included because they were either not germane or not preferred for your program. The firm names are listed in alphabetical order, with the brand labels and products listed after them. Many of these more-expensive items will be available only in better pharmacies or department stores.

Products for the Skin

Shaving Aids

Bethco (Burberrys)—After Shave Balm. (Lagerfeld)—After Shave Baume, Mousse a Raser, Protective Cream, Beard Softener.

Beecham (Hermes)—Aftershave Gel. (Jovan "Gambler")—After Shave Balm. (Lancaster)—Aftershave Conditioning Cream.

Henry N. Calisher (Capucci Pour Homme)—After Shave Balm.

Caron (Pour Un Homme)—After Shave Balm.

Chanel (Antaeus)—Moisturizing Shave Cream, Soothing Moisturizing Balm, Spray Talc. (Chanel For Men)—Shave Creme, After Shave Balm.

Jacqueline Cochran (Geoffrey Beene–"Grey Flannel")—Moisturizing Shave Cream, After Shave Balm. (Pierre Cardin)—After Shave Balm, Precision Shave Cream.

Colonia (Gucci Pour Homme)—After Shave Balm. (Kanon)—After Shave Balm.

Cosmair (Armani Pour Homme)—After Shave Balm. (Guy Laroche)—After Shave Balm. (Warner–"Chaps")—After Shave Balm. (Ralph Lauren Monogram)—After Shave Balm. (Polo)—After Shave Balm, Talc.

Dana—After Shave Soother, Shaker Talc.

Frances Denney (Adolfo For Men)—After Shave Balm.

Christian Dior (Eau Sauvage)—After Shave Balm, After Shave Moisturizer.

Faberge (Brut)—After Shave Cream Lotion, Soothing After Shave.

Fragrances Du Monde (De Viris)—After Shave Balm. (One Man Show)—After Shave Balm.

Fragrances Selective (Monsieur Carven)—After Shave Balm. (Vetiver)—After Shave Balm. (Marbert Man)—After Shave Soother, After Shave Cream, Pre-Shave Lotion.

Parfums Givenchy (Givenchy Gentleman)—After Shave Balm, Absorbent Talc. (Monsieur De Givenchy)—After Shave Balm, Talc.

Guerlain (Habit Rouge)—After Shave Creme.

Interface—Close Shave Formula.

Parfums Jacomo (Jacomo De Jacomo)—Shave Cream, After Shave Balm.

Jason Natural Products—Great Shave Mousse.

Jordache—After Shave Soother.

Key West Aloe—Brushless Shave Cream, Zele After Shave Gel. (K West)—Electric Pre Shave, After Shave Gel.

Calvin Klein (Calvin)—After Shave Balm.

Estee Lauder (Lauder For Men)—Shave Cream, Spray Talc, After Shave. (Aramis)—Super-Rich Shave Concentrate, Soothing Shave Cream, Shaving Crock w/Soap, Shaveplex Cream, Special Shaving Formula, Badger Shave Brush, Soothing After Shave, Pre-Shave Softener, Pre-Electric Lotion, Moisturizing After Shave. (Aramis 900)—Shave Cream. (Aramis 900 Herbal)—After Shave Soother. (Devin)—After Shave Soother. (JHL)—After Shave Balm, Cream Shave, Shave Soap, Brush Shave.

Prince Matchabelli (Matchabelli)—Soothing After Shave Balm.

Minnetonka (Roger & Gallet "L'Homme")—Shaving Cream, Talcum Powder.

Noxell (Noxzema) Shave Lather, Brushless Shave.

Paradise (Cruzan)—Aftershave Balm.

Puig/Barcelona (Quorum)—After Shave Balm. (Paco Rabanne "Paco For Men")—Shave Balm, Shave Cream, After Shave Soother.

. *Ben Rickert* (Bene)—After Shave Soother.

Charles of the Ritz (Yves Saint Laurent-Pour Homme)—After Shave Balm, Soothing After Shave, Shaker Talc.

Paul Sebastian—Pre-Shave Softener, After Shave Balm.

Shulton (Old Spice)—Pre-Electric Lotion, Shave Cream, Shave Mug w/Soap.

Parfums Stern (Oscar De La Renta–Pour Lui)—Cream Shave Vitale, After Shave, Balm Vitale.

Jan Stuart—Shave Cleanser, After Shave Toner, Night Cream/ Beard Softener.

Swank (Royal Copenhagen)—CEC Shave Lather, Blade Defense, CEC Shave Cream, Pre-Electric Shave, Pre-Shave Beard Softener, After Shave Balm, Shave Cream, Shave Brush.

Victor of Milano (Acqua di Selva)—After Shave Balm.

The Wilkes Group (Azzaro)—After Shave Balm.

Woods of Windsor (Woods of Windsor for Gentlemen)—Shave Mug/Soap, Badger Shaving Brush, After Shave Balm, Pre-Shave.

Skin Maintenance Aids

Bethco (Burberrys)—Soap, Bath/Shower Gel. (Lagerfeld)—Gel Pour Le Bain, Protective Cream, Moisturizing Bronzer, Soap Trio.

Dr. Babor Natural Cosmetics—Moisturizing Cream, Body Shampoo, Refreshing Mask.

Beecham (Lancaster)—Shower Gel, Bath Soap. (Vitabath-Zizanie)—Soap, Moisturizing Face Conditioner, Moisturizing Shower Gelee, Moisturizing Facial Scrub.

Beramic (Van Cleef & Arpels)—Soap, Emulsifier/Moisturizer, Shower & Bath Gel.

Henry N. Calisher (Capucci Pour Homme)—Soap. (Alain Delon) —Soap, Bath/Shower Gel.

Chanel (Antaeus)—Protein Skin Conditioner, Soap. (Chanel for Men)—Soap, Shower/Bath Gel, Hand Cream.

Jacqueline Cochran (Geoffrey Beene–"Grey Flannel")—Face Cream, Soap, Bath/Shower Gel.

Cosmair (Polo)—Soap, Moisturizer.

Delby (Sea Horse)—Bath Sponges. (The Disk)—Skin Care Buffer.

Fragrances Selective (Monsieur Carven)—Soap, Bath/Shower Gel. (Vetiver)—Soap, Bath/Shower Gel. (Marbert Man)—Soap, Night Line Smoother, Moisturizing Cream, Moisturizing Lotion, Tan Moisturizer, Face Mask, Face Exfoliant, Skin Control Stick.

Heitland International (Robert Ashley)—Moisture Cream, Tanning Cream.

Houbigant (Monsieur Houbigant Musk)—Soap, A Man's Moisturizer.

Interface—Work-Out Kit, Deep Cleanser, Toner, Day Moisturizer, Work-Out Mask, Herbal Scrub, Night Replenisher, Sun Bronzer, Body Hydratant.

Parfums Jacomo (Jacomo De Jacomo)—Soap, Skin Scrub, Body Shampoo, Hydro Actif Moisturizer.

Calvin Klein (Calvin)—Body Wash, Bath Bar, Skin Bronzer.

Estee Lauder (Lauder for Men)—Cleansing Bar, Face Tonic, Face Scrub, Comfort Lotion, Skin Repair Compound. (Aramis)—RNA Moisture Cream, All Year Bronzer, Body Care, Hand Cream, Soap, Body Shampoo, Muscle Soothing Soak. (Aramis 900 Herbal)—Soap, Body Shampoo. (Devin)—Country Soap, Country Body Shampoo, Face Conditioner, Country Hand/Body Moisturizer.

Puig/Barcelona (Paco Rabanne–"Paco For Men")—Soap, Sport Emulsion, Shower Gel, Facial Toner, Facial Scrub, Moisturizer, Basics Kit, Plus Kit.

Charles of the Ritz (Yves Saint Laurent–Pour Homme)—Facial Scrub, Face Protection Cream.

Paul Sebastian—Soap, Facial Toner, Moisturizer.

Shulton (Old Spice)—Skin Conditioner.

Jan Stuart—Day Moisturizer, Masque, Eye Cream, Honey/Almond Scrub, Body Moisturizing Mist.

Swank (Royal Copenhagen)—Deep Pore Cleanser, Cleansing Cream, Cleansing Lotion, Lip Relief, Bronzer, CEC Moisturizer, Eye Wrinkle Control, Facial Moisturizer.

Uniperf (Nino Cerutti–Pour Homme)—Soap, Lotion Moisturizer, Shower/Bath Foam Gel.

The Wilkes Group (Azzaro)—Soap, Body Shampoo, Face Moisturizer, Double-Action Cream, Tinted Face Bronzer.

Products for Problem Skin

ACNE SOAPS:
> *Bristol Myers*: Multi-Scrub (liquid or cream)
> *Cooper Labs*: Acnaveen
> *Stiefel Labs*: Acne-aid Detergent Soap
> *Westwood Pharmaceuticals*: Fostex

ACNE MEDICATIONS SOLD OVER-THE-COUNTER:
> *Dermik Labs*: Loroxide Acne Lotion
> *Cuticura-Purex*: Acne Cream
> *Revlon, Inc.*: Oxy-5 Acne Lotion
> *Vick Chemical Co.*: Clearasil Antibacterial Acne Lotion

PRESCRIPTION ACNE MEDICINES:
Dermik Labs: 5-Benzagel and 10-Benzagel
Steifel Labs: Benoxyl-5 and Benoxyl-10 lotions
Steifel Labs: Sulfoxyl Lotion, Regular and Sulfoxyl Lotion, Strong
Steifel Labs: Panoxyl-5 and Panoxyl-10 Gels
Texas Pharmaceuticals: Persa-Gel 5% and Persa-Gel 10%
Westwood Pharmaceuticals: Desquam-X 5 and Desquam-X 10 Gels.

Products for the Hair

Shampoos and Conditioners

Dr. Babor Natural Cosmetics—Shampoo.
Parfums Caron (Pour Un Homme)—Shampoo.
Chanel (Antaeus)—Shampoo. (Chanel For Men)—Conditioning Shampoo.
Jacqueline Cochran (Geoffrey Beene–"Grey Flannel")—Conditioning Shampoo. (Pierre Cardin)—Protein/Shampoo.
Cosmair (Polo)—Shampoo.
Fragrances Selective (Marbert Man)—Shampoo, Balsam Conditioner.
Parfums Givenchy (Givenchy Gentleman)—Gel Shampoo. (Monsieur De Givenchy)—Mild Shampoo.
Heitland International (Robert Ashley)—Shower Shampoo Gel.
Calvin Klein (Calvin)—Protein Shampoo.
Estee Lauder (Aramis)—Malt Enriched Shampoo, Malt Enriched Shampoo Concentrate, Malt Enriched After Shampoo, Malt Enriched Conditioner. (Aramis 900 Herbal)—Shampoo. (Devin)—Country Collagen Shampoo.
Minnetonka (Roger & Gallet)—Shampoo, Hair Conditioner.
Paradise (Cruzan)—Shampoo, Hair Conditioner.
Swank (Royal Copenhagen Classic)—Shampoo.
Victor of Milano (Acqua di Selva)—Liquid Shampoo.
The Wilkes Group (Azzaro)—Daily Hair Shampoo.
Woods of Windsor (Woods of Windsor for Gentlemen)—Shampoo.

There are countless other satisfactory shampoos on the market that don't carry the designation "for men only." They also exclude the special masculine packaging and the higher price tags. Here are a few of the better shampoos, most with additives to ease various hair problems:

Clairol, Inc.—Clairol Herbal Essence, Clairol Short and Sassy.
Alberto Culver Co.—Alberto Balsam Shampoo.
Helene Curtis—Everynight Balsam & Protein Shampoo.
Faberge, Inc.—Faberge Organics Pure Wheat Germ Oil & Honey Shampoo.
Mennen Company—Protein 21 pH Balanced Shampoo.
Owen Labs.—Ionax Shampoo for Oily Hair and Scalp, R-gen Protein Hair Repair Shampoo.
Pantene Co.—Pantene Shampoo for Fine or Thin Hair.

Dandruff Shampoos

Abbott Labs.—Selsun Blue.
Herbert Labs.—Vanseb Dandruff Shampoo with Protein.
Lederle Labs.—Zincon Dandruff Shampoo.
Owen Labs.—Iocon Shampoo Tar Gel Concentrate for Dandruff Control, Ionil T Nonionic/Cationic Therapeutic Dandruff Shampoo, Ionil Nonionic/cationic Therapeutic Dandruff Shampoo.
Proctor and Gamble—Head and Shoulders Shampoo.
Reedco, Inc.—Tegrin Medicated Shampoo.
Steifel Labs.—Polytar Shampoo.
Westwood Pharmaceuticals—Sebulex Medicated Shampoo.

Specialized Grooming Aids

Bristol Myers Co.—Vitalis Dry Texture for Men's Hair, Vitalis Clear Gel for Greaseless Hair Groom, Vitalis with V-7.
Jacqueline Cochran (Geoffrey Beene)—Styling Gel.
Alberto Culver Co.—Consort Hair Spray for Men.
Dana—Hair Gel.
Dep (Dep for Men)—Dry Styling Gel, Aerosol Hair Spray, Hair Spray.

Fragrances Selective (Merbert Man)—Hair Spray.

Johnson Products (Ultra Style)—Curls & Waves Kit, Wave Pomade.

Calvin Klein (Calvin)—Hair Fixative.

Estee Lauder (Aramis)—Malt Enriched Gel, Malt Enriched Thickener, Malt Enriched Hair Spray, Maltplexx Hair Gel.

Minnetonka (Roger & Gallet)—Supple Hair Fixative.

Woods of Windsor (For Gentlemen)—Hair Tonic.

This is, by no means, a complete list of every skin and hair care product on the market. For the most part, I have simply listed the newer men's products that might have escaped your attention. Inclusion on this list should not be construed as a personal endorsement. Consider this chapter a visual aid to help you locate the products that might work best for you. Again, experimentation is the best plan of action.

11

Common Sense

With deep apologies to the great patriot Thomas Paine, I think it's not altogether inappropriate to steal the title of his 1776 revolutionary tract for the concluding chapter of this book on skin and hair care. It is only common sense that the good looks and health of the skin and hair are ultimately dependent on the general health and working order of the entire body. I am not a medical doctor, so I am not going to usurp your time with boring theories that hint that you'll soon be able to outrun John McEnroe on the tennis court or whip "Refrigerator" Perry in a bout of arm wrestling. I do think it's important to remind you of general health rules that have a direct and decided impact on the condition of your skin and hair.

Diet

There'll be no long-winded recipes here that will direct you to the kitchen to whip up a repugnant repast of tasteless health foods. That time is better spent working on your personal grooming program. However, research has proved that the skin and hair can both be affected by a deficiency of certain vitamins, and diet can't be taken lightly. The food and drink we put into our bodies are both fuel and tonic. A standard, well-balanced diet will supply most of the important nutrients you need, but I'm aware that the pressure of work can make it tough to always eat properly. Vitamin supplements can be a great help. Vitamins and minerals that benefit skin and hair can also be found in such normal foods as fish, eggs, milk, cheese, cabbage and other leafy green vegetables, rice, grains, canteloupe, and even peanuts.

Obviously, if you have a cholesterol problem, you'll want to take it easy on the red meats and obtain your skin and hair helpers from other sources. Eating and drinking sensibly is the only true prerequisite for a healthy diet, even one designed to promote weight control. The use of too much salt, for example, should be avoided for a number of reasons: the sodium causes the body to retain too much water, it can contribute to high blood pressure, and research has proved that it adversely affects the hair. One scientific test indicated that "desalting" of the body arrested hair loss in males and in some cases appeared to reverse it. That particular experiment was not the breakthrough discovery it could have been because the subjects were desalted with the use of diuretics that had dangerous side effects. Suffice it to say that salt is no friend of any man worried about poor circulation or falling hair.

It's an unhappy fact that a man's concern about aging skin and hair usually arrives at the same time as he recognizes a need to start watching his waistline. Both problems can be treated at the same time with satisfactory results, but the key to that success depends on patience. Any weight reduction scheme that guarantees fast results is likely to destroy the good work you've been doing in restoring your skin and hair. Many of them induce dehydration that will send the indicator of your bathroom scale downward along with your skin and hair, sagging in the same direction because of an inadequate supply of natural moisture. Advice on diet comes at us every day from every direction. You can sum it all up in just two words: common sense.

Exercise

As humans were not devised to live by bread alone, they were also not created to be only flesh-and-blood money machines. Modern technology is making it increasingly clear that the days are limited when many of us—certainly in the United States—will be earning a living through muscles and sweat. The realization of that dream is already beginning to create a new problem. What is going to happen to that body with its intricate system of bone, muscle, tissue, and blood that was meant to be vigorously used?

There's a better than average chance that you are already employed in a job that takes a greater toll on your nervous system and the seat of your trousers than on your muscles. The current fitness craze in America was an inevitable and worthwhile byproduct of the new industrial revolution. Whatever your age or professional position, it is vital that you get adequate exercise to benefit your general health and the condition of your skin and hair. The facial exercises outlined earlier are excellent for toning the face, but you need regular amounts of vigorous physical exercise in order to keep the entire system functioning properly.

Anything you do that stimulates the circulatory system is going to help you live longer and look younger for as long as you live. Aerobic exercises are especially important in this regard, and, if you can't get into marathon running, at least bypass the limousine or taxi ride occasionally for brisk walks from office to business calls. If you're deskbound and have no time for visits to a health club, there are any number of simple exercises you can do at your desk (and even on the telephone) during your workday which will keep your skin and muscle tone young and healthy.

So your work calls for brains rather than muscle. So what? A good supply of the former will tell you that it's sinful to permit the deterioration of the latter. If you've abandoned the boyhood dream of looking like Charles Atlas instead of the ninety-seven-pound weakling, you should remember that a lack of proper exercise will also make your skin look like faded celery, and you'll end up with hair to match. Again, the bottom line is common sense.

Stress

There's almost no way we can avoid stress and stay in the mainstream of life as it is lived today, but it behooves us to give it our best shot. Some men actually thrive for a time on stressful emergency situations, otherwise, we wouldn't have happy firemen, policemen, test pilots, and so on. The hidden stress that most of us endure in our more mundane occupations can be even more insidious. It often makes its unhealthy presence known first in the most noticeable places: the face and hair. There is simply no doubt that stress can sneak up on us and undo much of what we have accomplished in our skin and hair care program.

Obviously, if there was any simple way of overcoming the effects of stress, none of us would suffer from it. A glass of wine or beer before dinner is one method, approved of even by many members of the medical establishment. But, as we have already learned, too much booze or a reliance on "recreational" drugs can also be destructive to the skin and hair, not to mention other vital parts of the body. There is plenty of evidence to support the theory that calculated use of a daily relaxation or meditation period, and strict adherence to it come hell or high water, can be an excellent escape valve.

A favorite sport, used as both a hobby and an exercise, can be another invaluable aid in helping you get away from it all. You may feel pressure lining up a four-foot putt or readying a second serve, but it will be a temporary and different kind of pressure from what you experience normally. That kind of activity will take your mind off the job and give you time to smell the roses. It's easier said than done, but set an alarm clock in your mind that will let you know when it's *your* time. "They" will see to it that you give them their full share of *company* time.

Odds and Ends About Hair and Skin

There are many practical tips that will help you preserve or regain a youthful face and hair that I skipped in the body of this book because they come under the heading of plain common sense. That being the case, this would seem the ideal space in which to list a few.

Sleep

No amount of cleaning, exfoliating, moisturizing, or other aids can prevent a droopy, haggard face if you don't get enough sleep. The amount needed varies from person to person, but it's almost impossible to get too much for the sake of your appearance.

Water

It's not only the single most important external aid in sound skin and hair care, but it's also a must ingredient in your daily diet. Like sleep, you can't get too much of it. Try to drink seven glasses of water per day, and up the ante on days when heat or exercise puts you in danger of dehydration.

Grimacing

Smiles and frowns are the greatest sculptors of deep lines in our kissers. Don't give up smiling, but be aware of the nonsmile crevices on your face, and discontinue the habit of facial contortion that carved them there.

Humidifiers

Dehydration is a constant menace to the health of skin and hair. There's a hidden indoor danger during the winter because so many heating systems rob our homes and offices of their normal humidity. A commercial humidifier or even a pan of water on the radiator can make a difference in the texture of your winter skin and hair.

"Starpower"

I've saved this tibit for the end because it seems a shame to waste an unscientific secret that so many Hollywood stars (especially Paul Newman) consider something of a "wonder drug" for good skin. I'll just label it "Ice is Nice." It can become a refreshing facial that you might enjoy at the end of your morning ritual. Fill the bathroom basin with clean. Cold tap water and lower the water temperature further by dipping in about two trays worth of ice cubes contained in a clean, porous cloth. When the water is really frigid, take a deep breath and hold your face under as long as possible. If your skin becomes uncomfortably cold, come up for air immediately. pat dry, spray your face with mineral water, and apply an invisible day moisturizer. I can't guarantee you'll look like Paul Newman, but you will be wide awake with tighter pores and you will have stimulated your circulation.

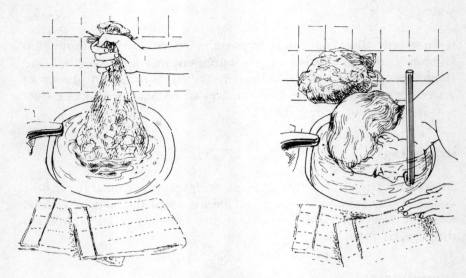

Ice water skin secrets

The Ball Is in Your Court

I made a deliberate effort in writing this book to avoid all references to a five-minute, thirty-day, or blah-blah plan that will return your skin and hair back to its youthful health and handsomeness. That sort of thing would look inviting in print, but it would also be (to put it kindly) misleading. The reality of the situation insists that any program aimed at rejuvenating your face and hair must include your patience as a principal ingredient.

You now possess the information and the techniques to complete the job that (I must assume) you were intent on starting. The rest is squarely up to you. You really can take years off the appearance of your skin and hair by taking advantage of what you have learned and investing a few extra minutes of your time each day to put that knowledge to work. The really important results of that effort are not going to be readily apparent the first day or the first week. I'm confident you will notice a surface improvement within a few days, but this program was designed to do far more than that. Dedicated adherence to it, on a daily basis, will allow you the confidence of knowing you look your best for the rest of your life.

Think young!

Index